Coronary flow reserve - measurement and application

BASIC SCIENCE FOR THE CARDIOLOGIST

1. B. Swynghedauw (ed.): *Molecular Cardiology for the Cardiologist.* Second Edition. 1998   ISBN 0-7923-8323-0

2. B. Levy, A. Tedgui (eds.): *Biology of the Arterial Wall.* 1999
    ISBN 0-7923-8458-X

3. M.R. Sanders, J.B. Kostis (eds.): *Molecular Cardiology in Clinical Practice.* 1999   ISBN 0-7923-8602-7

4. B.Ostadal, F. Kolar (eds.): *Cardiac Ischemia: From Injury to Protection.* 1999
    ISBN 0-7923-8642-6

5. H. Schunkert, G.A.J. Riegger (eds.): *Apoptosis in Cardiac Biology.* 1999
    ISBN 0-7923-8648-5

6. A. Malliani, (ed.): *Principles of Cardiovascular Neural Regulation in Health and Disease.* 2000   ISBN 0-7923-7775-3

7. P. Benlian: *Genetics of Dyslipidemia.* 2001   ISBN 0-7923-7362-6

8. D. Young: *Role of Potassium in Preventive Cardiovascular Medicine.* 2001
    ISBN 0-7923-7376-6

9. E. Carmeliet, J. Vereecke: *Cardiac Cellular Electrophysiology.* 2002
    ISBN 0-7923-7544-0

10. C. Holubarsch: *Mechanics and Energetics of the Myocardium.* 2002
    ISBN 0-7923-7570-X

11. J.S. Ingwall: *ATP and the Heart.* 2002   ISBN 1-4020-7093-4

12. W.C. De Mello, M.J. Janse: *Heart Cell Coupling and Impuse Propagation in Health and Disease.* 2002   ISBN 1-4020-7182-5

13. P.P.-Dimitrow: *Coronary Flow Reserve – Measurement and Application: Focus on transthoracic Doppler echocardiography.* 2002   ISBN 1-4020-7213-9

KLUWER ACADEMIC PUBLISHERS – DORDRECHT/BOSTON/LONDON

Coronary flow reserve - measurement and application:

Focus on transthoracic Doppler echocardiography

Paweł Petkow-Dimitrow, MD

2nd Department of Cardiology

Jagiellonian University

School of Medicine

Kraków

KLUWER ACADEMIC PUBLISHERS
Boston / Dordrecht / London

Distributors for North, Central and South America:
Kluwer Academic Publishers
101 Philip Drive
Assinippi Park
Norwell, Massachusetts 02061 USA
Telephone (781) 871-6600
Fax (781) 681-9045
E-Mail: kluwer@wkap.com

Distributors for all other countries:
Kluwer Academic Publishers Group
Post Office Box 322
3300 AH Dordrecht, THE NETHERLANDS
Telephone 31 786 576 000
Fax 31 786 576 474
E-Mail: services@wkap.nl

 Electronic Services < http://www.wkap.nl >

Library of Congress Cataloging-in-Publication Data

A C.I.P. Catalogue record for this book is available
from the Library of Congress.   ISBN 1-4020-7213-9

Coronary Flow Reserve – Measurement and Application: Focus on transthoracic
Doppler echocardiography by Pawel Petkow-Dimitrow

***The Publisher offers discounts on this book for course use and bulk purchases.
For further information, send email to melissa.ramondetta@wkap.com.***

To my wife Ula

CONTENTS

ACKNOWLEDGEMENTS

I am indebted to Professor Andrzej Beręsewicz, MD for his valuable comments and suggestions.

All echocardiograms were recorded in the Echocardiographic Laboratory 2nd Department of Internal Medicine, Jagiellonian University School of Medicine in co-operation with Marek Krzanowski, MD in whom I heartily acknowledge the long time co-work, support and invaluable suggestion in preparing this monograph.

I greatly appreciate helpful comments of Stefan Chłopicki, MD

Special thanks are due to my teacher Professor Jacek S. Dubiel, MD

I am especially indebted to Wacław Kuś for his technical help.

Finally, I need to say a word of thanks to Zyta Turek for her linguistic contribution to this monograph.

LIST OF ABBREVIATIONS

Cx – circumflex coronary artery
EDV – endothelium dependent vasodilatation
EIDV – endothelium independent vasodilatation
FFR – fractional flow reserve
LAD – left anterior descending coronary artery
NO – nitric oxide
PET – positron emission tomography
PTCA – percutaneous transluminal coronary angioplasty
RCA – right coronary artery

INTRODUCTION

Coronary flow reserve is an important functional parameter to understand the pathophysiology of coronary circulation. Coronary flow reserve measurement is used to assess epicardial coronary stenoses or to examine the integrity of microvascular circulation. An appreciation of coronary physiology is an integral part of clinical decision-making for cardiologists treating patients with coronary artery disease. The pioneering research efforts of Dr Lance Gould, who explored the relationship between the anatomic severity of a stenosis and its flow resistance (59;60) , have been transferred to clinical practice (94;194). In the absence of stenosis in epicardial coronary artery, the coronary flow reserve may be decreased when coronary microvascular circulation is compromised by arterial hypertension with or without left ventricular hypertrophy, diabetes mellitus, hypercholesterolemia, or other diseases.

Several techniques have been established for measuring coronary flow reserve. However, these techniques are either invasive (intracoronary Doppler flow wire), highly expensive and scarcely available (Positron Emission Tomography - PET) or semi-invasive and causing patient discomfort (transesophageal Doppler echocardiography), thus their clinical use is limited. Because of the clinical importance of coronary flow reserve there is a need for a simple, noninvasive, repeatable and inexpensive tool capable of this functional evaluation. This monograph focuses on the assessment of coronary flow reserve using transthoracic Doppler echocardiography – the technique fulfilling the above-mentioned criteria. Transthoracic Doppler echocardiography has become a popular tool evolving from a research to diagnostic technique applied in everyday practice. In one of the numerous institutions performing transthoracic Doppler echocardiography to measure coronary flow reserve almost 1000 patients were examined, thus demonstrating the usefulness of this method in various clinical settings (111). In the present monograph PET is additionally described since this method is considered as the "gold" standard for noninvasive assessment of coronary flow reserve.

Transthoracic Doppler echocardiography is used to evaluate increases in coronary blood flow velocity, which may be a result of endothelium-independent or endothelium-dependent vasodilatation in response to an appropriate stimulus. The increase in coronary blood flow mediated by endothelium-independent vasodilatation is defined as the classical coronary flow reserve. However, a nearly similar increase in coronary blood flow may be induced by acetylcholine (which is used to test endothelium-dependent vasodilatation), but only in those subjects in whom major factors predisposing to endothelial dysfunction (hypercholesterolemia, arterial hypertension, diabetes mellitus, and smoking) are absent. In contrast, endothelium-dependent vasodilator response is impaired or even reversed to vasoconstrictor pattern in the presence of these factors. Pharmacological and non-pharmacological treatment may restore normal coronary vasodilator response, however the number of studies documenting the beneficial effect of therapy on the improvement or restoration of endothelium-dependent vasodilatation is small due to limited availability of PET imaging. A wider use of transthoracic Doppler echocardiography as a noninvasive technique to evaluate endothelium-dependent vasodilatation may provide an insight into this issue. Original studies from our institution in a group of patients with hypertrophic cardiomyopathy contribute to exploring this issue (137-143) Pharmacological and non-pharmacological correction of endothelial dysfunction is especially important in view of the fact that coronary endothelial dysfunction predisposes to adverse cardiovascular events in medium- and long-term follow-up studies (159;169)

At first sight the monograph seems to be addressed to a small group of specialists. However, it is intended to provide a broad view of multifactorial coronary flow impairment. This may be the case when a patient presents with chest pain despite insignificant coronary stenosis or even absent atherosclerotic changes in coronary angiogram. Invasive intracoronary Doppler examination reveals coronary flow reserve impairment in 60% of such patients. The patients in this subgroup usually have one or more of the following diseases: diabetes mellitus, hypercholesterolemia, syndrome X, myocardial hypertrophy (complicating arterial hypertension, hypertrophic cardiomyopathy, aortic stenosis), coronary microvascular disease (vessel wall remodeling) in arterial hypertension without myocardial hypertrophy. Intracoronary Doppler to measure flow velocity is not widely available and for this reason noninvasive transthoracic Doppler echocardiography to estimate coronary flow reserve is a useful tool, especially in patients with anginal pain and hemodynamically insignificant coronary stenosis.

In presence of coronary artery stenosis, understanding the functional impact of stenosis is important for clinical decision making (for example to refer or defer patients with intermediate stenosis to PTCA). The treatment of patients with moderate stenoses is challenging, and coronary flow reserve measured distally to stenosis is helpful to define the hemodynamic significance of the lesion. Transthoracic Doppler echocardiography might also be useful in subjects with significant epicardial arterial stenosis. In patients undergoing PTCA noninvasive serial monitoring of coronary flow reserve may help in detecting restenosis.

Chapter 2 explains that one of the most important problems in clinical decision making is the lower limit of normal coronary flow reserve (mediated by endothelium-independent vasodilatation). The threshold value has not been definitely specified, yet. In this context limitations of various techniques estimating coronary flow reserve have been discussed. With these limitations in mind investigators continue their effort for a search of more precise methods. Accordingly, new coronary flow reserve-derived indices (fractional flow reserve and relative coronary flow reserve) obtained from invasive measurements, have been briefly described. Additionally, the results of large invasive studies (DEBATE, DESTINI), in which coronary flow reserve was a guided tool (complementary to lumenology) for stenting strategy have been reported in brief.

The choice of an appropriate diagnostic tool and a stimulus of vasodilatation is of major practical importance, which has been discussed in the last chapter. For instance, fairly uncomfortable semi-invasive transesophageal echocardiography combined with dipyridamole, which may produce unpleasant side effects, is not well-tolerated by patients.

Summing up, this monograph will discuss the current concepts of the pathophysiology of coronary circulation and methods to measure coronary vasodilatation (focusing on noninvasive transthoracic Doppler echocardiography) and provide practical insights for patient management. In particular, the monograph intends to show [1] how endothelium-independent coronary flow reserve can be measured noninvasively, [2] how endothelium-dependent vasodilatation can be effectively estimated and [3] in which clinical settings these measurements are applicable.

Chapter 1

BLOOD FLOW REGULATION IN CORONARY CIRCULATION

Introduction

Blood flow (Q) in the coronary circulation depends on the coronary perfusion (driving) pressure (ΔP) and the resistance (R) offered by the coronary vascular bed. The relationship between these parameters is described by the modified Ohm's law as follows:

$$Q = \frac{\Delta P}{R}$$

Coronary perfusion pressure is the difference between mean aortic pressure and right atrial pressure. As in normal conditions right atrial pressure is low, it is assumed that perfusion pressure is approximate to mean aortic pressure. In the steady state, coronary blood flow is maintained at a relatively constant level in the range of coronary perfusion pressure approximately from 40 to 130 mmHg. This phenomenon is referred to as autoregulation of coronary blood flow. This ability to maintain unchanged coronary blood flow in the face of fluctuating perfusion pressure within autoregulation range results from the fact that changes in pressure are balanced by changes in coronary vascular resistance. In contrast, when resistance is minimized by a vasodilator, coronary circulation escapes from autoregulation and pressure-flow relationship becomes linear. The difference between the baseline (autoregulated) coronary blood flow and the coronary blood flow after maximal vasodilatation is referred to as coronary flow reserve. Coronary vascular resistance, in turn, is regulated by several control mechanisms listed below:

- Myogenic control of vascular tone (a regulatory component contributing to autoregulation)
- Extravascular compressive forces due to increased intramural myocardial pressure (the contributing role of this component also enhances with increasing left ventricular diastolic pressure compressing particularly the subendocardial layer)
- Anatomically determined vascular diameter
- Rheological properties of blood (this component plays a minor role and refers to the relationship between changes in blood viscosity and resistance)

Mathematically vascular flow resistance is expressed by the formula of Poiseuille:

$$R = \frac{8\mu L}{\pi r^4}$$

where r- is the radius of the vessel, μ- viscosity of the blood, L- length of the vessel.

In the coronary circulation with stable blood viscosity, the only element, which may change dynamically, is the vessel's radius. The vascular resistance-radius relationship is inverse and because of the fourth power effect even slight changes in the radius are translated into marked changes in resistance.

1.1   Structure of coronary vascular system

The coronary arterial tree consists of four basic segments presented schematically in Figure 1-1. Epicardial arteries give off small transmural penetrating arteries (vessel diameter: 300-100 μm), which branch in the myocardial layers. These branches are defined as arterioles (100-10 μm), terminating as capillary vessels (<10 μm), directly supplying myocardial cells. Each of these segments produces various resistance to coronary blood flow. Large epicardial coronary arteries play a minor role in the regulation of coronary vascular resistance and act principally as conductance (conduit) vessels. Most of the resistance, which opposes coronary blood flow, arises from resistance arterioles. The resistance is manifest by decreased coronary perfusion pressure (Figure 1-2.). The percent distribution of the length and resistance of individual segments of the coronary vascular tree has been summarized in Table 1-1. In the presence of a significant epicardial stenosis, coronary perfusion pressure decreases at the site of stenosis and subsequently trans-stenotic pressure gradient is generated (Figure 1-3.).

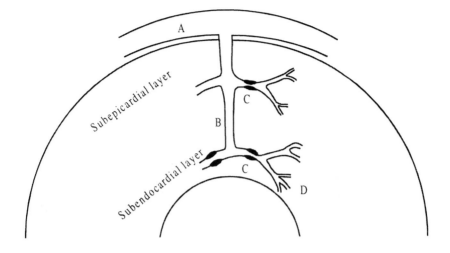

Figure 1-1. Segmental arrangement of coronary vascular bed: A- epicardial artery B- small transmural (perforating) artery C- arterioles D- capillary vessels

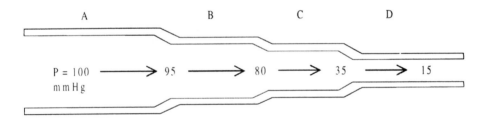

Figure 1-2. Sequential decrease in coronary perfusion pressure in consecutive segments of coronary vasculature. The largest fall in perfusion pressure occurs in resistance arterioles.

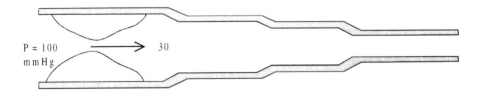

Figure 1-3. Significant reduction of coronary perfusion pressure distally to stenosis in epicardial artery (trans-stenotic pressure gradient is 70 mmHg).

1.2   Regulation of coronary blood flow

Vascular tone regulating resistance is under balance between counteracting (vasodilating versus vasoconstricting) factors, which affect smooth muscle in coronary arteries. Vascular tone is regulated by several mechanisms including myogenic, metabolic, endothelial and neural control and extravascular compressive forces (14;35;55;85;86;114;165). Additionally, humoral factors (endothelin, angiotensin) provoke vasoconstriction (66;168). Importantly, coronary arterioles appear to have specialized regulatory, diameter-specific elements along their length (Table 1-1.) (14;34;114;167). As for endothelial regulation it plays a decidedly more important role in the microcirculation than in large (conductance) coronary arteries (Table 1-1.).

Table 1-1. Morphologic and functional characteristics of coronary arterial bed

	A. Large epicardial arteries	B. Medium-sized and small arteries	C. Arterioles	D. Capillaries
Diameter	>1000 µm	1000-100 µm	100-10 µm	<10µm
% of total resistance	5%	15-25% 400-100 µm	50-60%	20%
% length of coronary bed	5-10%	15-25%	60-75%	
	Regulatory mechanisms responsible for coronary vasomotion			
Metabolic: Adenosine ? K^+_{ATP} channels ?			+++ (>30 µm)	+
Endothelial: NO	+	+++ (80-150 µm)		+
Myogenic:		+	+++ (30-80 µm)	

Clinically available techniques do not allow for the measurement of small vessel diameter. For this reason a change in their caliber is concluded from changes in coronary blood flow in the epicardial artery.

1.2.1   Myogenic autoregulation of coronary blood flow

The principle of myogenic flow regulation is that vascular smooth muscle cells react to increased intramural pressure by contraction and oppositely, when intramural pressure declines, vascular smooth muscle cells relax. The consequent autoregulation of resistance tends to return blood flow toward the steady-state despite perfusion pressure. fluctuation within the range of autoregulation approximately from 40 to 130 mmHg. The regulatory role of myogenic autoregulation to maintain unchanged coronary blood flow (14;34;84-86;114) is illustrated in Figure 1-4., displaying the pressure-flow relationship in the autoregulated steady-state as a plateau with a slightly positive slope (18). Beyond the autoregulation range only extremely low and high coronary perfusion pressure induces a linear increase in coronary blood flow (84;127). Autoregulation occurs only in coronary vessels with preserved vascular smooth muscle tone. In contrast, when resistance is minimized by a vasodilator, the pressure-flow relationship significantly changes.

1.2.2   The concept of coronary flow reserve

After maximal vasodilatation (hyperemia) coronary blood flow is no longer autoregulated and varies linearly with coronary perfusion pressure (Figure 1-4.). The difference between the coronary blood flow corresponding to the autoregulation plateau under baseline conditions and the coronary blood flow after maximal vasodilatation is termed as coronary flow reserve (14;55;74;98;127). Coronary flow reserve is expressed as the ratio of maximal (hyperemic) to baseline coronary blood flow. Coronary flow reserve depends on various factors decreasing its value (see details in chapter 2). The routinely used stimuli to test coronary flow reserve induced via endothelium-independent vasodilatation (EIDV) are adenosine or dipyridamole. Intracoronary papaverine was used previously.

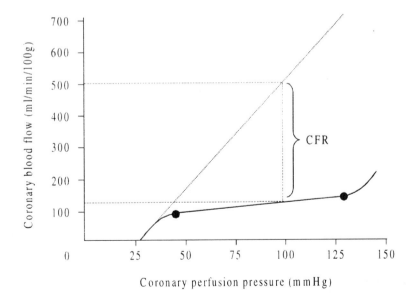

Figure 1-4. Pressure-flow relationship in coronary circulation. Baseline (autoregulated) coronary flow is marked with a solid line. Large circles indicate the lower and upper limits of autoregulation range (approximately 40 and 130 mm Hg). Dotted line indicates maximum vasodilatation. Coronary flow reserve (CFR) = 500/125 = 4,0

1.2.3   Endothelium-independent coronary vasodilatation (EIDV)

The scheme in Figure 1-5. shows that adenosine acts on the last stage of the vasodilative cascade without the involvement of the endothelium.

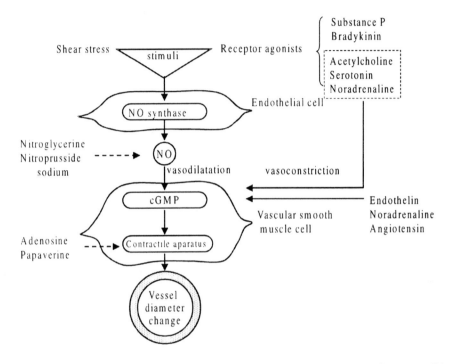

Figure 1-5. A schematic representation of the signal transduction cascade responsible for vascular tone regulation. Normally, vasodilatation counterbalances vasoconstriction. In endothelial dysfunction the delineated receptor agonists cannot stimulate NO (nitric oxide) -dependent vasodilatation and they act as vasoconstrictors directly on vascular smooth muscle. For simplification, only more frequently used vasoactive substances have been shown.

Dipyridamole vasodilating effect is mediated through adenosine. Dipyridamole induces vasodilatation indirectly by inhibition of the re-uptake of adenosine by vascular endothelial cells. Because of this effect, the onset and offset of the action of dipyridamole are unfavorably prolonged (see Table 5-2. in section 5.1.1.). The exogenous and endogenous (increased by dipyridamole) adenosine stimulates a group of purinergic receptors A_1, A_2, A_3. The activation of A_1 receptor causes undesirable side effects: slowing of the heart rate and conduction through the atrioventricular node. Receptors A_{2A} and A_{2B} are found on the surface of smooth muscle cells and their activation causes vasodilatation in most vascular beds including coronary circulation. Adenosine relaxes mainly small resistance arterioles. The proposed mechanism of adenosine action is that activation of A_2 receptors causes stimulation of cyclic AMP production leading to decreased uptake of calcium by the sarcoplasmic reticulum and hence subsequent smooth muscle relaxation and vasodilatation. At high concentration during intracoronary infusion (12 to 54 µg) adenosine acts via EIDV pathway, as it crosses the endothelial barrier and directly stimulates receptors A_2 in the smooth muscle. At lower concentration adenosine may elicit mild endothelium-dependent vasodilatation (EDV).

1.2.4 Endothelium-dependent coronary vasomotion

Since the pioneering work of Furchgott and Zawadzki (52) the endothelium has been recognized as a major regulator of vascular homeostasis. Endothelial cells, as the inner lining covering blood vessels, are strategically located between circulating blood and vascular smooth muscle cells. The monolayer of endothelial cells is able to transduce blood-borne signals and sense mechanical forces within the lumen. Subsequently, endothelium as a signal transducing organ regulates vascular tone through the generation and release of various vasoactive substances (55;113;126;184;191). The functional integrity of endothelium is crucial for the maintenance of vascular homeostasis in the following processes:
- Regulation of vasomotor tone and proliferation of vascular smooth muscle,
- Platelet activation, adhesion and aggregation
- Thrombogenesis and fibrinolysis
- Monocyte/macrophage rolling, adhesion, transmigration and retention in the subendothelial space (initiation of atherosclerosis)

1.2.4.1 Stimulation by receptor agonists
Endothelial cells produce and release numerous substances affecting the vascular tone. Of these vasoactive substances the best known is nitric oxide (NO), a mediator with strong vasodilating properties. NO may be released under the influence of various substances stimulating on appropriate receptors on the surface of the endothelium (acetylcholine, substance P, serotonin, noradrenaline, bradykinin) (Figure 1-5.) (52;55;112;113;126;147;148;200). These main agonists in human studies are infused intracoronarily in pharmacological tests to evaluate (EDV) in the coronary circulation. Noradrenaline is not given intracoronarily but its endogenous release is stimulated in cold pressor test. In case of endothelial dysfunction acetylcholine, serotonin, noradrenaline cannot stimulate the production of NO, but unopposedly constrict smooth muscle in the vascular

wall (Figure 1-5.). A net effect is paradoxical vasoconstriction, which was first described by Furchgott and Zawadzki in their pioneer study (52), in which they stimulated endothelial-denuded artery using acetylcholine.

1.2.4.2   Role of shear stress

Another important NO stimulator is the frictional force generated by blood flow shearing the surface of the endothelium. This force, referred to as shear stress (τ) is directly related to blood flow according to the formula:

$$\tau = \frac{4Q\mu}{\pi r^3}$$

where Q- blood flow, μ- blood viscosity, r- vessel radius

In vessels with constant blood flow the endothelium using NO synthase produces a basic amount of NO, which exerts tonic vasodilating effect (148). A proof of the endothelium-dependent vasodilatation effect of NO is the fact that NO synthase inhibitor (inducing NO deficit) causes vasoconstriction.

One could say that shear stress is a natural stimulus to release NO due to increased coronary blood flow. In the normal coronary circulation increased blood flow is induced by the following physiological factors (metabolic stress tests): exercise test (47;58), tachycardia (rapid atrial pacing) (129;147;153;155), cold pressor test (128;198-200) and mental test (197). The mechanism by which these tests operate is the increased myocardial oxygen demand, which forces a compensatory increase in coronary blood flow, on condition that the flow limiting factors (endothelial dysfunction, vasospasm, atherosclerotic stenosis) are absent.

1.2.5   Coronary endothelial dysfunction

The EDV mechanism involves a cascade of processes displayed in Figure 1-5. Most clinical tests evaluating endothelial function consist in the measurement of arterial diameter or blood flow (reflecting the microcirculation resistance) after various interventions stimulating endothelial NO generation. These tests measure in fact the final stage of the cascade of vasomotor response to stimulation. Therefore the mere statement of abnormal vascular response is not sufficient to diagnose endothelial dysfunction. It should be remembered that apart from decreased NO production, the same vasomotor impairment may be a result of impaired contractility of smooth muscles, their decreased sensitivity to cyclic guanosine monophosphate (cGMP), defect of guanylate cyclase, or impairment of NO diffusion. Therefore an important element of each examination evaluating EDV is a control test, which measures additionally the effects of exogenous NO donor (nitroglycerine, sodium nitroprusside, acting only on the level of epicardial arteries because in microvessels there is no enzyme necessary to metabolize nitroglycerine into its active form i.e. NO) and substances directly relaxing smooth muscle cells via EIDV (adenosine, dipyridamole, papaverine). In practice, endothelial dysfunction is diagnosed when EDV is impaired and EIDV is preserved or impaired to a lesser degree than EDV. A measure of endothelial dysfunction is the decreased ratio of EDV/EIDV (see also section 1.2.6)

1.2.5.1   Mechanisms of vasodilator endothelial dysfunction

It is known that vasodilator endothelial function is related mainly to NO, which as a key-factor competes with vasoconstrictive substances (angiotensin, endothelin, noradrenaline) (Figure 1-5.). The endothelial dysfunction may be a derivative of the following abnormalities (Table 1-2.) (55;113;183):

Table 1-2. The mechanisms of endothelial dysfunction due to loss of NO bioavailability:

• Decreased NO production
(e.g. due to deficient of tetrahydrobiopterin, a cofactor for NO synthesis)
• Increased activity of endogenous inhibitors of NO synthase
(e.g. accumulation of asymmetric dimethyl arginine ADMA)
• Increased NO degradation as a result of oxygen radicals overproduction
• Cholesterol-mediated reduction of transcription or stability of messenger RNA encoding the NO synthase
• Impaired diffusion of NO to smooth muscle cells

Summing up, NO plays several fundamental cardioprotective roles including the control of endothelium-dependent vasodilatation, leukocyte adhesion, expression of adhesion molecules, platelet aggregation, inhibition of vascular growth. Thus, impairment of endothelial NO bioavailability has become an attractive target of therapeutic interventions. As regards diagnosis of endothelial dysfunction, a number of circulating surrogate markers of endothelial dysfunction and vascular inflammation has been extensively studied over the past few years. The following soluble markers are proposed: cellular adhesion molecules, C-reactive protein, von Willebrand factor, endothelin, tissue plasminogen activator.

1.2.5.2   Stages of endothelial dysfunction

In normal conditions a stimulus testing endothelial function evokes vasodilatation. In the presence of endothelial dysfunction the ability to vasodilate is impaired or even lost, and in advanced stages of dysfunction counterbalancing mechanisms inducing vasoconstriction begin to dominate. It has been found that endothelial dysfunction progresses with increasing

severity of atherosclerosis (128;129;198;200). Figure 1-6. shows gradual
progression of endothelial dysfunction. The scheme is simplified by
averaging vasomotor response to various stimuli (or various doses of the
stimulus) testing EDV.

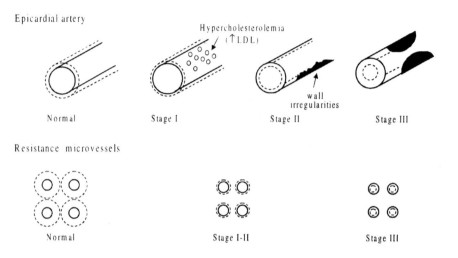

Figure 1-6. A schematic sequel of endothelial dysfunction: I - initial stage (angiographically
normal artery), II - intermediate stage (vessel wall irregularities, minimal atherosclerotic
changes), III - advanced stage with significant atherosclerotic stenosis (details in text).

In an epicardial coronary artery, an early stage of endothelial dysfunction is
featured by decreased or abolished EDV, and with increasing dysfunction
there is even pathological reversal of vasodilatation to vasoconstriction.
Further progression of endothelial dysfunction in the epicardial artery
(usually coexisting with significant stenosis) is manifest by marked
vasoconstriction in response to a stimulus. Within the microcirculation,
where vascular resistance mainly resides, the pathological vasomotor
response resulting from endothelial dysfunction consists mainly in lower
augmentation of coronary blood flow under stimulation as compared with
the controls. In advanced dysfunction, which accompanies marked epicardial
artery stenosis, coronary blood flow decreases under stimulation
(128;129;156;169;199;200). Particularly important is the phenomenon that
the loss of EDV occurs in early atherosclerosis, even prior to its detection by
coronary angiography. (Figure 1-6. Stage I). In these circumstances
endothelial dysfunction is a valuable marker of the hidden onset of
atherosclerosis (112;120;193;200). This loss of NO bioavailability (reduced
synthesis and/or accelerated breakdown of NO) is related to risk factors for
atherosclerosis.

1.2.5.3   Risk factors predisposing to endothelial dysfunction

It is important that treatment modifying risk factors of endothelial dysfunction (55;113;183;191) (summarized in Table 1-3.) improves EDV, even though there is no angiographic evidence of the regression of atherosclerosis (13).

Table 1-3. Risk factors of endothelial dysfunction:

• hypercholesterolemia
• hypertriglyceridemia
• arterial hypertension
• diabetes mellitus
• cigarette smoking
• post-menopausal estrogen deficit
• deconditioning
• hyperhomocysteinemia
• aging
• congestive heart failure

Endothelial dysfunction may be a very dynamic process. Rapidly increasing triglycerides in blood within several hours after a fat meal may induce endothelial dysfunction manifest by decreased EDV (166). An equally rapid may be the regression of endothelial dysfunction with improved EDV, after LDL-cholesterol apheresis (175).

Endothelial dysfunction has a systemic nature (3). Thus, impaired EDV (due to the presence of the above mentioned risk factors) applies not only to coronary but also peripheral circulation (3). Brachial artery has been used as a surrogate target to measure endothelial dysfunction, because this artery is very easily accessible, which provides an opportunity of repeated imaging by ultrasonography. The plethysmographic methods may additionally assess peripheral microcirculation. Using these methods and stimulus of post-occlusive reactive hyperemia we may serially monitor the effects of modification of endothelial dysfunction risk factors. Long-term prevention has shown that the reduction of elevated blood pressure (ACE-inhibitors), cholesterol (statins), glucose and cessation of smoking, estrogen replacement therapy in postmenopausal women and increased physical activity improve or restore EDV in peripheral circulation (2;55;113;183;191). However, brachial and myocardial circulation are very different in terms of flow and resistance patterns, metabolic regulation, receptor population contributing to humoral regulation and microvascular architecture (189). In this view, it is highly desirable to abandon the surrogate target (brachial artery) to focus on coronary circulation, which is now accessible using transthoracic Doppler echocardiography.

1.2.6   The endothelium-dependent / endothelium-independent
              vasodilatation ratio

The diagnosis of endothelial dysfunction consists in the statement that EDV is impaired and EIDV is preserved or impaired to a lesser degree than EDV. A measure of endothelial dysfunction is thus a decreased ratio of EDV/EIDV. Coronary flow reserve is routinely assessed by infusion of adenosine or dipyridamole, vasodilators acting via EIDV. In humans with angiographically normal coronary circulation, coronary flow reserve tested with these vasodilators is characterized by increased coronary blood flow by 150-500% on average (31;76). Similar values have been shown after acetylcholine, which by inducing EDV, increases coronary blood flow by 200-350% on average, and in single cases even by 500% (31;76;148). It should be emphasized that such high values have been obtained only in selected subjects, with partially excluded risk factors for endothelial dysfunction (hypertension, diabetes mellitus, partially hypercholesterolemia). According to the quoted studies (31;76) the EDV/EIDV ratio is around 0,90. Because of the selection criteria these studies were performed in a small group of subjects with chest pain as an indication to invasive study and unfortunately including smokers. For this reason the normal EDV/EIDV ratio in healthy subjects is not known. It seems reasonable to suggest that the more complete elimination of risk factors for endothelial dysfunction through selection of study subjects makes this value close to 1,0. It is possible that in totally healthy subjects without the risk factors of endothelial dysfunction, the value of EDV is equal to EIDV. This hypothesis is difficult to verify for ethical reasons, because acetylcholine is given only intracoronarily, which entails invasiveness. The EDV/EIDV ratio decreases in patients with endothelial dysfunction risk factors, but without significant stenosis in epicardial arteries in the following way: in patients without myocardial ischemia at scintigraphy it is 0,56 (201). In case of myocardial perfusion defect, this ratio is further decreased to 0,23 (201). These data and additional findings where the EDV/EIDV ratio was not calculated (listed in Table 1-4.) suggest that the decrease in EDV precedes the decrease in EIDV.

An indirect confirmation of this suggestion is the disproportion between the values proposed as lower limits of normal EDV [blood flow increased by 50% after acetylcholine (63;169)] and for EIDV [blood flow increased by 150% after adenosine (63)]. This decreased value for EDV relative to EIDV seems to result from the fact that among the patients with chest pain and without significant stenosis by coronary angiography there were subjects with endothelial dysfunction risk factors (63), which caused this disproportion.

Table 1-4. Comparison between EDV and EIDV in relation to stress test results

		EDV	EIDV	
Zeiher et al.(201)	Negative scintigraphy	199% *	389%	(papaverine)
	Positive scintigraphy	80% *	351%	(papaverine)
Hasdai et.(62)	Negative scintigraphy	42% *	220%	(adenosine)
	Positive scintigraphy	-11% *	200%	(adenosine)
Cannon et al.(25)	Positive ExT, negative DOB	179% #	432%	(adenosine)
	Negative ExT, negative DOB	169% #	402%	(adenosine)
All study groups were heterogeneous (patients had various risk factors for endothelial dysfunction), * selected data obtained during infusion of an identical, intracoronary dose of acetylcholine 10^{-6} mol/L were presented for correct comparison, # different dose of acetylcholine i.e. median acetylcholine dose 100 µg/min (range 3 to 300 µg/min), ExT-exercise test, DOB- dobutamine stress echocardiography				

Suwaidi et al (169) proposed the following classification of endothelial dysfunction tested by acetylcholine: moderate – blood flow velocity increased from 0% to 50% (reduced EDV) and advanced – decreased blood flow velocity below the value at rest (vasoconstrictor response of the microcirculation). Another way of interpreting the results of EDV is to verify the EDV values by comparing them with the results obtained in the control group consisting of healthy volunteers. The use of noninvasive methods to assess coronary flow reserve in healthy volunteers is obligatory.

1.2.7 The prognostic value of coronary vasodilator endothelial dysfunction

Impaired EDV has a prognostic value in patients with non-significant or even absent stenosis at baseline coronary angiography. It has been shown (159) that endothelial dysfunction (vasoconstrictor response of epicardial artery to acetylcholine or cold pressor test) predicts the occurrence of adverse cardiovascular events: unstable angina, myocardial infarction, revascularization procedures at follow-up (a mean of 7,7-years). Suwaidi et al. (169) also confirmed the unfavorable prognostic role of endothelial dysfunction (assessed cumulatively at epicardial and microvascular level) measured as changes in coronary blood flow after acetylcholine, even in a shorter 28-month follow-up. In their study (including 3 subgroups) cardiovascular complications occurred in a subgroup of patients with vasoconstrictor response to acetylcholine (EDV<0%) manifested by a decrease of coronary blood flow by 38% (in average). In patients in whom coronary blood flow significantly increased after acetylcholine (EDV>50%) adverse effects did not occur. Interestingly, free from adverse effects were also patients from the intermediate group defined by an acetylcholine test result [i.e. 50%>EDV>0%, consequently these patients had a small increase in coronary blood flow by 24,8±2,8% concomitantly with slight epicardial vasoconstriction by −13,7±2,8%]. EIDV was not reduced and was similar in all three subgroups studied by Suwaidi (169). In contrast, Schachinger et al. (160) preliminarily reported that papaverine- or adenosine-induced EIDV increases are predictive for adverse cardiovascular events.

Chapter 2

THE RANGE OF NORMAL VALUES FOR CORONARY FLOW RESERVE AND LESION-SPECIFIC PHYSIOLOGICAL MEASUREMENTS

Introduction

In peripheral circulation oxygen extraction from perfusing blood is as low as 25%. In contrast, the amount of oxygen extracted by myocardium during a passage of blood through the coronary circulation is very high i.e. 70% in resting conditions. Consequently, during stress testing myocardial oxygen extraction may increase only slightly. For this reason myocardial oxygen supply depends mainly on the efficiency of the coronary vasodilatation augmenting the coronary blood flow to match the increasing myocardial metabolic demand. Pharmacological vasodilatation increasing coronary blood flow in relation to baseline value determines coronary flow reserve.

Despite great research efforts, a clear-cut threshold value for coronary flow reserve, to determine the functionally significant severity of coronary stenosis is not definitely established. The proposed threshold values of coronary flow reserve for clinical decision making range from as low as 1,8 up to 3,0. The lower limit of normal value is so important and intriguing that Voci et al. (189) named it magic number of 2,0 or 2,5. Currently it seems justified to regard as unequivocally abnormal the value below 2,0 (blood flow increased by 100%), whereas normal values are those exceeding 3,0 (blood flow increased by 200%). Practical implications from determination of the borderline coronary flow reserve between 2,0 and 3,0 are now being tested in clinical studies, especially on provisional stenting strategy. The equivocal lower limit of normal coronary flow reserve (range 2,0-3,0) corresponds to a large scatter of coronary flow reserve values in reference groups. This phenomenon is most probably a result of a multitude of measurement techniques and heterogeneity of control groups, which is a consequence of non-uniform entry and exclusion criteria (some control subjects may have microvascular vasodilator dysfunction reducing coronary flow reserve). Coronary flow reserve depends on a number of factors limiting maximal vasodilatation (other than epicardial stenosis) or increasing resting coronary blood flow, which in turn also reduces coronary flow reserve. In order to reduce these limitations two novel measurements have been introduced, namely relative coronary flow reserve and fractional flow reserve.

2.1   The lower limit of normal coronary flow reserve

2.1.1   Comparison of measurements using different methods

When testing EIDV in normal coronary vascular bed, coronary blood flow increases usually by 3 to 5 times relative to baseline value. An important issue from the practical viewpoint is to define the lower limit of normal coronary flow reserve (Table 2-1.).

Table 2-1. Comparison of coronary flow reserve measurements using different methods in groups considered as reference (control) groups.

Number of patients	Method	CFR	Reference
17 (HTX)	D.I.	5,0±0,3	(119)
26 (HTX)	D.I.	5,2±1,3	(30)
18 (young subjects)	PET	4,1±0,9	(41)
22 (elderly subjects)	PET	3,0±0,7	(41)
28	PET	3,2±1,2	(110)
31	PET	3,8±2,1	(82)
56	PET	3,4±1,4	(181)
19	D.TTE	3,7±0,7	(69)
26 (athletes)	D.TTE	5,9±1,0	(69)
Subjects with chest pain despite angiographically normal coronary arteries (patients with hypercholesterolemia, hypertension, diabetes mellitus, smoking were included)			
85	D.I.	2,8±0,6	(93)
CFR – coronary flow reserve; D.I. – invasive intracoronary Doppler, D.TTE- noninvasive transthoracic Doppler echocardiography, HTX- routine assessment of coronary flow reserve early after heart transplantation			

The normal limits may depend on a number of factors, including the methodology of measurement. Table 2-1. summarizes the results of selected studies taking into account the most numerous study groups. Three techniques are compared: invasive and noninvasive Doppler measurements and noninvasive PET. It is noteworthy that Doppler technique is used to measure local coronary flow velocity, whereas PET measures myocardial perfusion, both global and regional. A wide scatter of the values can be seen both within a given technique and between individual studies. An especially high standard deviation in a PET study by Iida et al. (82) is noteworthy. Such a wide scatter is probably a result of PET limitations, discussed in more detail in section 4.3.

2.1.2   Enrolment criteria for recruited subjects

Before we define the normal value of coronary flow reserve, we should identify appropriate subjects for recruitment to reference groups. In noninvasive studies we may recruit any subjects who give informed consent to examination. The perfect candidate is a healthy volunteer with neither cardiovascular sings and symptoms nor risk factors for endothelial dysfunction/coronary artery disease. In contrast, invasive studies are performed in subjects with chest pain, implying that coronary microvascular vasodilator dysfunction may limit coronary blood flow despite normal epicardial arteries. Two studies (63;150) demonstrate that such coincidence is quite frequent. Bearing in mind this limitation it has been proposed by Baumgart et al (6) that in invasive measurements normal limits of coronary flow reserve may be derived only from highly selected subjects according to the following restricted criteria:
– truly normal epicardial arteries confirmed by intracoronary ultrasound examination
– age <50 years
– asymptomatic subject (additionally I propose an obligatory absence of risk factors for endothelial dysfunction)

All these criteria can be met in patients early after heart transplantation (in later postoperative follow-up coronary flow reserve may decrease due to transplant vasculopathy), if the heart was harvested from a healthy young trauma victim. Following this suggestion Table 2-1. contains invasive data collected exclusively from patients undergoing control examinations after heart transplantation. Importantly, in these highly selected subjects coronary flow reserve markedly exceeded the cut-off value 3,0 being the closest to the highest value obtained in athletes.

The recruitment of reference subjects with normal epicardial arteries verified by intracoronary ultrasound is crucial as indicated by the following example. Positive exercise scintigraphy, primarily evaluated as false positive due to angiographically normal coronary vessels may frequently turn out to be true positive as control intracoronary ultrasound reveals vascular lesions (188). It is noteworthy that reduced coronary flow reserve was a fairly good predictor of "soft lesions" non-visualized by coronary angiography (188).

Baumgart (6) proposed a criterion of age below 50 years, which is reasonable, as PET in younger subjects revealed a significantly higher coronary flow reserve than in the elderly (see Table 2-1.). The investigators (41) demonstrated that coronary flow reserve reducing with age was a result of increased coronary blood flow at rest, whereas maximal blood flow remained relatively stable despite aging. Only in subjects above 70 years of age maximal coronary blood flow is also reduced. Thus according to Baumgart et al (6) the lower limit of normal coronary flow reserve is 3,0 for subjects up to 50 years of age.

Another information in Table 2-1., which requires comment, is reduced coronary flow reserve below 3,0 in patients with chest pain despite normal coronary vessels but including subjects with hypertension, hypercholesterolemia, diabetes and smoking (93). Such patients had been frequently recruited to invasive studies, which was criticized (115). When comparing the results obtained by Kern et al. (93) with other findings cited in the Table 2-1. it is obvious that such patients are characterized by coronary flow reserve, which is lower than in other groups. Reduced coronary flow reserve in patients with stenocardia but without significant lesions in epicardial coronary vessels is a problem encountered in a large group of patients studied invasively. In a large study by Hasdai et al. (63) 58,5% of patients had reduced coronary flow reserve exclusively in the microcirculation. Reduced EDV was observed in 29,2% patients, EIDV in 11,3% patients, whereas mixed dysfunction was found in 18% patients. A relatively low proportion of subjects with EIDV dysfunction was probably related to the fact that the cut-off value for normal coronary flow reserve (EIDV) was lowered in this study from 3,0 to 2,5. However, in another study, coronary flow reserve (EIDV) <2,5 was more frequent (in 60% of patients) in women with stenocardia and normal coronary arteries (150).

The highest value was observed in athletes, which was partially associated with decreased coronary blood flow at rest (69). This reduction may derive from a slower heart rate at rest in trained athletes and consequently lower myocardial oxygen demand. Bradycardia is one of the adaptation mechanisms related to regular training.

2.2   Factors limiting coronary flow reserve

Coronary flow reserve may be limited generally by two groups of abnormalities (59;60;74;98) (Table 2-2., Figure 2-1.):

Table 2-2. Two groups of factors limiting coronary flow reserve:

1. Increase of baseline coronary blood flow due to increased myocardial oxygen demand as a result of:
•   tachycardia
•   increased myocardial contractility
•   myocardial hypertrophy
2. Decrease of maximal (hyperemic) coronary blood flow by:
•   epicardial coronary artery stenosis
•   wall thickening (remodeling) of resistance arterioles
•   reduced density of arterioles
•   cardiomyocyte hypertrophy
•   perivascular fibrosis
•   interstitial fibrosis
•   endothelial dysfunction
•   increased blood viscosity
•   elevated left ventricular diastolic pressure increasing extravascular compressive forces and resistance (particularly in subendocardial layer).

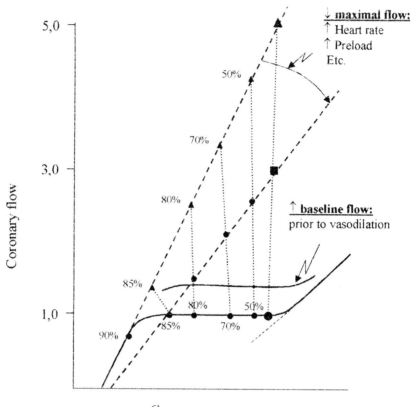

Coronary pressure

Figure 2-1. Complexities of the flow reserve concept. See text for details. [from Klocke FJ. Measurements of coronary flow reserve: defining pathophysiology versus making decisions about patient care. Circulation 1987;76:1183-1189. Lippincott Williams & Wilkins (reproduced with permission).

2.2.1   Stenosis of epicardial coronary artery

Epicardial stenosis decreases coronary perfusion pressure distally to stenosis site. The trans-stenotic pressure gradient is generated because of the loss of kinetic (flow) energy to viscous friction, turbulence, and flow separation. The degree of trans-stenotic pressure fall is related not only to increased percent of stenosis but also to flow rate as described by curvilinear (exponential) pressure-flow relationship of the particular lesion resistance (97) (see Figure 2-2.). The mathematical formula describing pressure-flow relationship is complex, and in a simplified form (55) it is presented with an additional scheme (see Figure 2-3.).

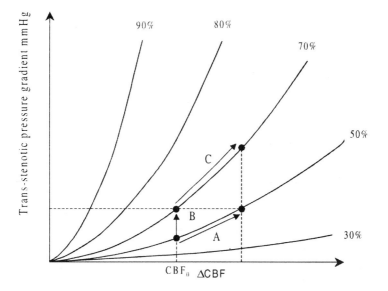

Figure 2-2. Relation between pressure reduction across a stenosis and coronary flow through the stenosis. Relations are shown for concentric stenoses of 30, 50, 70, 80 and 90 percent internal diameter. (modified from Klocke FJ: Measurements of coronary blood flow and degree of stenosis: Current clinical implications and continuing uncertainties. Newsletter of the Council on Clinical Cardiology of the American Heart Association. Vol. 7, No 3, 1982, reproduction with permission), A- pressure gradient increase due to slight flow augmentation (ΔCBF) despite only 50% stenosis, B- pressure gradient increment (similar as in situation A) with increasing degree of stenosis despite unchanged baseline flow (CBF_0), C- significant increment of pressure gradient despite slight flow augmentation (ΔCBF) in 70% stenosis.

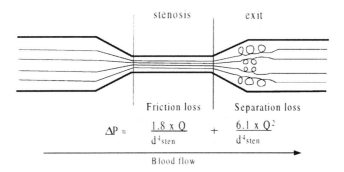

Figure 2-3. Energy losses across a stenosis (d sten- minimal diameter of stenosis lumen). The pressure gradient due to friction losses within stenosis (ΔP) is directly proportional to blood flow (Q), whereas separation losses at the exit to the stenosis due to formation of eddies increase with blood flow square (Q^2). Separation losses predominate at high blood flows (modified from Ganz P and Ganz W: Coronary blood flow and myocardial ischemia. In: Braundwald et al. „Heart disease" W.B. Saunders 2001;1100, reproduction with permission.

The first fraction accounts for viscous friction between layers of blood at the stenotic site leading to frictional energy losses. The second fraction reflects energy losses when the "pressure energy" of normal arterial flow is transferred first to the kinetic energy of high-velocity flow and then, at the exit from stenosis, to turbulent energy of distal flow eddies (separation losses due to disturbed laminar flow). As flow increases, separation losses, which increase with the square of the flow, become increasingly prominent. Augmentation of coronary flow induced by vasodilator or increasing myocardial oxygen consumption (metabolic stress test) is associated with elevation in trans-stenotic pressure gradient (Figure 2-2.), and reduction in post-stenotic perfusion pressure.

Accelerated reduction of coronary flow reserve in case of coronary artery stenosis >70% (Figure 2-1.), is a result of exponential gradient pressure-flow relationship (Figure 2-2.) (97). As stenosis increases, exponential relationship becomes steeper (Figure 2-2.). In approximately 90% stenosis, minimal augmentation of coronary flow induces rapid increase in trans-stenotic pressure gradient, immediately exhausting post-stenotic coronary flow reserve (Figure 2-1.). A second important conclusion from the curvilinear pressure-flow relationship is that not only the degree of stenosis but also augmented coronary blood flow increases trans-stenotic pressure gradient. The exponential fashion of the relationship explains why in the presence of intermediate stenosis (40-70%) perfusion pressure distally to the stenotic site may decrease significantly (due to increased trans-stenotic pressure gradient) (Figure 2-2.). This may happen for instance with a significant increment of coronary flow in response to increased myocardial oxygen demand induced by arterial hypertension complicated by left ventricular hypertrophy and superimposing tachycardia. In this example several factors increasing coronary blood flow (see Table 2-2.) are combined to produce the summation effect which may provoke myocardial ischemia in absence of significant epicardial stenosis. Summing up, the target of treatment may not only be widely recognized mechanical dilation of the stenosis but also pharmacological intervention to decrease high velocity of coronary blood flow. A recent study on metoprolol (15) and verapamil (140) effects on coronary flow velocity may be a good example of this pharmacological approach.

2.2.2   Transmural reduction of coronary flow reserve

Assessment of regional coronary flow reveals marked spatial heterogeneity of coronary flow reserve across the myocardial wall. The highest value of coronary flow reserve is measured in the subepicardial layer. Due to transmural reduction, coronary flow reserve in the subendocardial layer is significantly lower (also due to elevated left ventricular diastolic pressure increasing extravascular compressive forces). As a result of this transmural distribution, coronary flow reserve is exhausted first in the subendocardial layer (74) (Figure 2-4.). The lower limit of autoregulation is unfavorably shifted to the higher value of coronary perfusion pressure in the subendocardial layer as compared with the subepicardial layer (i.e. 55-65 mm Hg versus 30-40 mmHg, respectively) (14) (Figure 2-4.). According to Hoffman (74) the reduction of global coronary flow reserve from 4,0 to 2,0 could be associated with the loss of reserve in part or all of the subendocardium. Because of subendocardial vulnerability to ischemia, Hoffman suggested (74) that coronary flow reserve as 2,5 or even 3,0 is potentially damaging to the subendocardium. This theory supports the postulation that coronary flow reserve only above 3,0 is normal.

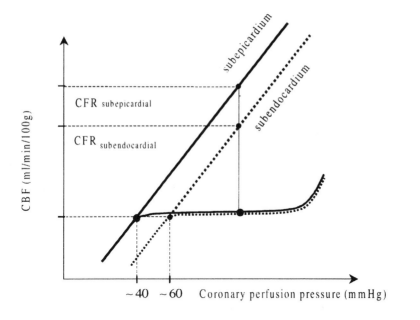

Figure 2-4. Transmural distribution of coronary flow reserve (CFR); CFR subepicardial > CFR subendocardial

2.3 A new index of functional severity of stenosis: lesion-specific physiological measurements

Epicardial stenosis and microcirculation abnormalities may coexist and cumulatively decrease the value of coronary flow reserve. From the practical point of view, it is essential to separate the detrimental effect of these two components. Unfortunately, an abnormal coronary flow reserve cannot differentiate which of the two components is responsible for flow impairment (Figure 2-5.). The unequivocal cutoff value for clinical decision making (i.e. conservative treatment, optimal PTCA with or without stenting) has not been defined despite great effort of investigators working in this field. Fractional flow reserve (FFR) and relative coronary flow reserve are new stenosis-specific measurements particularly useful for functional assessment of stenosis severity.

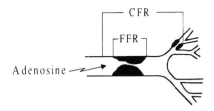

Figure 2-5. Coronary flow reserve reflects cumulative effects of epicardial and microvascular abnormalities. FFR measures the stenotic-specific effect independently of microvascular abnormalities.

2.3.1   Fractional flow reserve

Fractional flow reserve (FFR) is a newly developed concept of a pressure-derived estimate of coronary blood flow particularly useful for stenosis-specific physiological measurements (Figure 2-5.) (8-10;145). The formula for FFR calculated after adenosine infusion is as follows:

$$FFR = \frac{\text{mean post-stenotic coronary pressure}}{\text{mean pre-stenotic coronary pressure}}$$

FFR is defined as the maximal blood flow to the myocardium in the presence of a stenosis in the supplying coronary artery, divided by the theoretical normal maximal flow in the same distribution. This index represents the fraction of the normal maximal myocardial flow that can be achieved despite the coronary stenosis. In hemodynamically insignificant stenosis, perfusion pressure distal to stenosis is close to pre-stenotic perfusion pressure. As a result FFR is close to 1, which is the maximal value. With the increasing degree of stenosis the trans-stenotic pressure gradient also increases, and distal pressure decreases (see Figures in section 3.2.1). In patients with moderate coronary stenosis, FFR appears to be a practical index of the functional assessment of stenosis severity and the need for coronary revascularization (10;145). FFR is related to the ischemic potential of a stenosis. Patients with FFR>0,75 had no signs of myocardial ischemia during stress testing and did not require PTCA during conservative treatment at 2-year follow-up (8;145). The especially important application of FFR measurement concerns patients with an intermediate left main coronary artery stenosis (40-60%). In this particular case of equivocal left main coronary artery disease the measurement of FFR is useful in deciding whether or not to proceed to bypass surgery (9). In patients with FFR>0,75 coronary bypass surgery may be deferred and conservative (medical) approach with regular follow-up used instead. Importantly, the FFR value was closely correlated with cross-sectional area of left main coronary artery measured by intracoronary ultrasound, which is a much more precise parameter than artery diameter assessed in coronary angiography (personal communication Legutko J. and Dudek D.).

Although FFR seems independent of microvascular vasodilator dysfunction or changing hemodynamics, the magnitude of flow increase during maximal vasodilatation still influences FFR.

2.3.2 Relative coronary flow reserve

Baumgart et al. (6) rightly proposed that an indication to perform PTCA should be not only decreased absolute, post-stenotic coronary flow reserve < 3,0 but also decreased relative coronary flow reserve. Relative coronary flow reserve is a ratio of post-stenotic reserve in the target vessel to reserve in a nonstenosed reference vessel. Impaired relative coronary flow reserve indicates that coronary flow reserve in the stenosed vessel is lower than coronary flow reserve in the reference vessel regarded as normal (5;6). This adjustment of coronary flow reserve to the reference vessel allows for theoretical elimination of a possible vasodilator dysfunction in coronary microcirculation, as a cause of additional reduction in coronary flow reserve superimposing on the flow-limiting effect of epicardial artery stenosis. The normal value of relative coronary flow reserve is 1, whereas proposed values reflecting hemodynamically significant stenosis are listed in Table 2-4. (see section "2.4.3 Summary" at the end of chapter). The relationship between the value of relative coronary flow reserve and inducibility of myocardial ischemia during stress testing has been studied most extensively. In patients with relative coronary flow reserve >0,75 the signs of myocardial ischemia were not observed during either echocardiographic (48) or scintigraphic stress tests (50). Measurements of relative coronary flow reserve may be useful in detecting microvascular-derived stunning of the myocardium (Table 2-3.) supplied by a coronary artery undergoing PTCA.

Table 2-3. Microvascular-derived myocardial stunning is associated with limited maximal coronary flow in response to vasodilator infusion because of the following microvasculature obstructing factors:

- Humoral: release of vasoconstrictive substances from endothelium (endothelin, thrombin),
- Thrombogenic: aggregating plates at the site of the balloon injury with subsequent peripheral microembolisms
- Mechanical: microembolisms caused by atherosclerotic plaque fragmentation during PTCA

The cardiac enzymes (creatine kinase and cardiac troponin T) are proposed as surrogate markers of embolic myocardial injury. Cardiac marker elevation is associated with the reduction of relative coronary flow reserve (65;67), indicating periprocedural embolization originating from atherothrombotic debris (after plaque fragmentation) with microvascular obstruction and myocardial injury. Postprocedural relative coronary flow reserve <0,78 has been independently found predictive of the elevation of enzymatic marker of myocardial injury despite angiographically successful PTCA (67).

It should be remembered that the measurement of relative coronary flow reserve is precise only on condition that the severity of microcirculatory impairment is comparable in the vascular bed of target and reference vessel. This condition cannot be always met because of regional variation (heterogeneity) in coronary flow reserve between various segments of myocardial wall (74).

2.4   Application of coronary flow reserve measurement

Coronary flow reserve measurements are useful to assess: (a) severity of epicardial stenosis or (b) microvascular vasodilator dysfunction (small resistance vessel disease). An abnormal coronary flow reserve precisely assesses these two components only if they occur separately. In the assessment of epicardial stenosis, coronary flow reserve measurement is helpful in the following clinical settings:

– functional assessment of moderate stenosis (to refer for or defer coronary intervention)
– complementary role for making decision about stent implantation after PTCA (coronary flow reserve guided optimal PTCA).

Coronary flow reserve measurement allows for detecting microvascular vasodilator dysfunction in cardiological diseases manifested by stenocardia despite angiographically normal coronary artery [e.g. syndrome X, arterial hypertension (particularly complicated by myocardial hypertrophy), hypertrophic cardiomyopathy, myocardial hypertrophy due to severe aortic valve stenosis]. Additionally coronary flow reserve measurement is valuable in evaluating effects of pharmacological treatment in the above mentioned clinical settings (see chapter 3).

2.4.1 Coronary flow reserve in relation to stress-induced myocardial ischemia

From the practical viewpoint functional assessment of stenosis is associated with defining the degree of reduced coronary flow reserve, which corresponds to myocardial ischemia inducibility during stress testing (19;42;87;123). Coronary flow reserve < 2,0 has been found to predict myocardial ischemia in scintigraphy with high sensitivity and specificity (19;42;87;123). In a large study DEBATE the best cut-off value was 2,1 for coronary flow reserve in relation to outcome of exercise test (144). In another study (174) it was the same value of 2,1; which best differentiated patients with positive and negative dobutamine echocardiography stress test. In contrast, Zeiher et al. (201) showed that in all patients with positive scintigraphic test, coronary flow reserve significantly exceeded 2,0 (>100% increase in coronary blood flow), (see table 1-4. in section 1.2.6)

2.4.2 Decision making in coronary artery intervention

Invasive measurement of coronary flow reserve plays a complementary role to coronary „lumenology" for decision-making concerning physiological end points for coronary interventions. Apart from angiographic (anatomical) assessment, physiologic guidance of an intervention with intracoronary flow velocity measurement is a new concept to optimize the PTCA results. A Doppler-guided angioplasty approach has been evaluated in 3 multicenter trials: DESTINI-CFR (Doppler Endpoint Stent International Investigation of Coronary Flow Reserve), DEBATE I and II (Doppler End Point Balloon Angioplasty Trial, Europe) and FROST (French Optimal Stent Trial). These studies assessed whether a provisional, Doppler-guided approach produces clinical outcomes as beneficial as a primary or mandatory stent approach. Post-PTCA coronary flow reserve < 2,5 [DEBATE I, II (163;164)] or even a lower value < 2,0 [DESTINI (45)] was proposed as an indication for stenting. An intermediate value of 2,2 was proposed in FROST (49).

2.4.3 Summary

Table 2-4. summarizes the currently proposed lower limits of coronary flow reserve and its derivatives, as well as advantages and disadvantages of the three measurement methods.

Table 2-4. Comparison of absolute and relative coronary flow reserve and FFR

	CFR	RCFR	FFR
Independent of hemodynamic changes	-	+	+
Independent of microcirculation abnormalities	-	+**	+
Useful in multivessel CAD	+	-	+
Unequivocal normal values	>3,0	1	1
Unequivocal abnormal values	<2,0	0,65< [29;187]	0,75< [29;145]
Minimal value of CFR as an endpoint for PTCA DEBATE DESTINI FROST	 2,5*# 2,0*# 2,2*#	0,75-0,88 [5;64;92]	0,90 [10]
CAD- coronary artery disease, CFR- coronary flow reserve, RCFR- relative coronary flow reserve, * velocity-derived coronary flow reserve, ** on condition of homogeneity of microcirculatory vasodilatation # combined with morphological assessment of residual, postprocedural stenosis using intracoronary ultrasonography			

As the body of experience continuously grows the above cited minimal value of coronary flow reserve used as an end point for PTCA should be regarded as preliminary. For instance in a recent study (64) in a smaller group of patients (150 subjects) the best cut-off value for coronary flow reserve was 2,86 indicating the threshold below which the patients experienced death, myocardial infarct or restenosis within 6 months after PTCA.

Chapter 3

APPLICATION OF NONINVASIVE DOPPLER ECHOCARDIOGRAPHIC MEASUREMENT OF CORONARY FLOW RESERVE

Introduction

The preceding chapter described the application of coronary flow reserve measured by means of invasive techniques, which are of limited use. This chapter will focus on noninvasive tools used to assess coronary flow reserve in a wide spectrum of clinical settings. At present two noninvasive techniques are predominantly applied: Doppler echocardiography (transthoracic imaging is the technique, which develops most dynamically) and PET. Transthoracic Doppler echocardiography is rapidly gaining appreciation and it has become a popular tool evolving from a research to diagnostic technique applied on a large scale in everyday practice. In one of the numerous institutions performing transthoracic Doppler echocardiography (111), almost 1000 measurements of coronary flow reserve have been made in various cardiovascular diseases and using various pharmacological agents: vasodilators (dipyridamole, adenosine) and dobutamine, which increases myocardial oxygen demand.

Figure 3-1. shows a coronary angiogram (3-1a.) and schematic representation (3-1b.) of the LAD. Additionally the position of the transducer and orientation of the imaging plane to visualize the distal LAD are presented. In first studies echocardiography was used to assess the velocity of blood flow in the LAD according to the following concept. Transesophageal echocardiography visualized blood flow in the proximal LAD, whereas transthoracic echocardiography in the distal LAD.

A   B

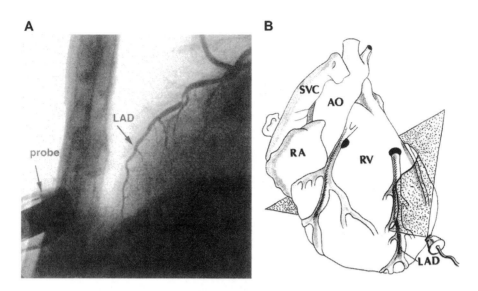

Figure 3-1. a) Coronary angiogram demonstrating the relative relation of the transthoracic probe to the LAD. (from Hozumi et al. Noninvasive assessment of significant left anterior descending coronary artery stenosis by coronary flow velocity reserve with transthoracic color Doppler echocardiography. Circulation 1998;97:1557-62, Lippincott Williams & Wilkins, reproduced with permission; *1b).* Artist's drawing illustrating transducer beam orientations to LAD. LV indicates left ventricle; SVC, superior vena cava; AO, aorta; RA, right atrium; and RV, right ventricle (from Caiati C et al. New noninvasive method for coronary flow reserve assessment: contrast- enhanced transthoracic second harmonic echo Doppler. Circulation 1999;99:771-8, Lippincott Williams & Wilkins, reproduced with permission).

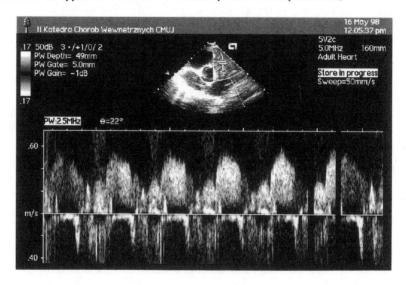

Figure 3-2. Spectral Doppler coronary blood flow by sampling in LAD.

The development of the transthoracic imaging technique (exploring various transducer beam orientations) extended the possibilities of imaging blood flow in the LAD to include its mid-portion and proximal segment (20;22;103). The examples of spectral Doppler recordings of coronary flow velocities in LAD are presented in Figure 3-2. According to the most recent reports, coronary flow reserve can be measured in the Cx (177) and RCA (107;189).

However, measurements of coronary flow reserve in the proximal LAD present some disadvantages limiting universal use of transesophageal Doppler echocardiography. Coronary flow reserve measured only in the proximal LAD is reliable for the assessment of the microcirculation on condition that there is no stenosis in further portions of the LAD and all important branches of the LAD are normal. In this situation coronary flow reserve is not limited on the level of epicardial artery and microcirculation abnormalities may be reliably evaluated in numerous patients with anginal pain despite angiographically normal coronary arteries (for instance syndrome X, arterial hypertension, hypertrophic cardiomyopathy, myocardial hypertrophy complicating severe aortic stenosis). In contrast, in the presence of stenosis, post-stenotic reserve is much more accurate than pre-stenotic reserve in assessing residual vasodilator capacity of the vascular bed subtended to a narrowed coronary artery. In fact, coronary flow reserve measured in regions with branches proximal to the lesion is pseudo-normalized and, thus, is diagnostically unreliable because flow is concurrently assessed for regions of varying vasodilator reserve, hence reflecting a weighted average of these potentially disparate zones (21). Figure 3-3. shows a diagram explaining this situation.

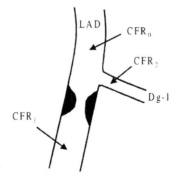

$$CFR_2 > CFR_0 > CFR_1$$

Figure 3-3. Substitutional measurement of CFR proximally to stenosis (CFR0) overestimates CFR1 distally to stenosis site, CFR0 is weighted average of CFR1 and CFR2 (in LAD branch), where CFR2 is normal. Dg-1 first diagonal branch.

Summing up, the measurement of coronary flow reserve in LAD by means of Doppler echocardiography may be divided from the practical point of view into:

– measurement of coronary flow reserve in the microcirculation with normal epicardial vessels (transthoracic and transesophageal echocardiography is useful here)

– measurement of post-stenotic coronary flow reserve in stenosed epicardial artery (transesophageal echocardiography is useless, unless the lesion can be visualized directly in the proximal segment and coronary flow reserve can be measured below the stenotic site).

As regards the transthoracic Doppler assessment of coronary flow reserve in the RCA we are able to measure the coronary flow velocity in proximal RCA and in its distal branch i.e. right posterior descending artery (see also section 4.1.2.1). Due to the fact that most relevant RCA stenoses are located proximal to the crux cordis the assessment of coronary flow reserve in the right posterior descending artery usually provide post-stenotic values.

PET is used to image perfusion of any myocardial region, which allows for unlimited measurement of coronary blood flow in the vascular bed of all coronary arteries: LAD, Cx and RCA. PET has however several limitations, which will be discussed in detail in section 4.3.

3.1   Microvascular vasodilator dysfunction

3.1.1   Hypercholesterolemia, hypertension, smoking, diabetes mellitus

The major factors predisposing to endothelial dysfunction and simultaneously to coronary artery disease include arterial hypertension, hypercholesterolemia, smoking, diabetes mellitus. In these situations EIDV may also be impaired. Noninvasive measurements of EDV and EIDV are performed in these clinical conditions, especially to verify therapeutic outcomes. In arterial hypertension, both EDV and EIDV have been found to be impaired in the coronary circulation (101;117;135) and pharmacotherapy (ACE-inhibitors, verapamil) may improve these parameters (117;135). Hypercholesterolemia has also been found to reduce EDV and EIDV, whereas hypolipidemic treatment (statins) efficiently abolishes this abnormality (61;80;161). As far as smoking is concerned the duration of the habit and intensity of smoking are directly correlated with the severity of endothelial dysfunction in coronary vessels (23). In diabetic patients noninvasive technique has also been found useful in detecting reduced coronary flow reserve (44). All the above-mentioned studies were performed using PET, however, recently transthoracic Doppler echocardiography has been successfully used in these clinical settings. Accordingly, coronary flow reserve decreased after a single high-fat meal in young healthy men (77), after 30 minute of passive smoking (133), in postmenopausal women (72) and in diabetic patients in whom the reduction of coronary flow reserve was inversely related to degree of diabetic retinopathy (124). Coronary flow reserve was $3,11\pm0,53$ in no retinopathy patients, $2,67\pm0,55$ in patients with simple retinopathy and $2,03\pm0,34$ in patients with proliferative retinopathy (124). From the therapeutic point of view, it is possible to monitor beneficial effects of statin (51) and estrogen replacement therapy on coronary flow reserve (72). Also, hypoglycemic therapy in diabetic patients is associated with the improvement of coronary flow reserve (125).

3.1.2 Vasculopathy in transplanted heart

Coronary artery disease of the allogenic heart transplant may develop in as many as 30% of patients within the first year after transplantation. It is believed that this specific type of coronary artery disease develops from immunological and non-immunological endothelial injury, with the loss of its integrity (186). As a result vasomotor dysfunction involves both the microcirculation and epicardial arteries (100). This type of generalized vasculopathy develops at various rates and with varying intensity after heart transplantation, and for this reason noninvasive monitoring of its progression seems especially valuable (100).

3.1.3 Hypertrophic cardiomyopathy

Coronary circulation in hypertrophic cardiomyopathy is characterized by a significant microvascular vasodilator dysfunction (termed as small vessel disease) despite usually normal epicardial coronary arteries. Available reports document a marked reduction of coronary flow reserve after dipyridamole - an agent inducing EIDV (37;56;110;122;136;162). Previously, the main noninvasive technique for measuring coronary flow was PET or transesophageal echocardiography. Apart from the reduction of global coronary flow reserve it has been found that dipyridamole in hypertrophic cardiomyopathy induces subendocardial ischemia due to transmural (horizontal) steal of blood from the underperfused subendocardium at the cost of increased flow in the subepicardial layer (37;56;110). Preliminary studies have shown that reduced coronary flow reserve is an unfavorable prognostic factor (28). In hypertrophic cardiomyopathy coronary microcirculation abnormalities (combined with marked hypertrophy) may be so advanced that the administration of dipyridamole reduces coronary blood flow below the initial value (172). As a result coronary flow reserve paradoxically falls below 1,0 (172). According to the authors this phenomenon occurs probably via the mechanism defined as vertical steal of blood from the LAD (perfusing hypertrophied septum) at the cost of increased flow in the competing Cx, which supplies the nonhypertrophied free wall.

In previous invasive studies, EDV was not precisely examined in patients with hypertrophic cardiomyopathy (26;27;81;99;104;132). The results of pharmacological (acetylcholine) or metabolic stress (rapid atrial pacing) testing suggested the impairment of EDV. However, these studies had certain limitations, because both stimuli were not used to study EDV but to another purpose (acetylcholine to provoke vasospasm and pacing to induce myocardial ischemia). These studies were performed mainly in patients with stenocardia as an indication for invasive coronary angiography. Personal studies using transthoracic echocardiography (137-141) due to their noninvasiveness included a broader spectrum of patients: asymptomatic, mildly symptomatic and with dyspnea as the dominant symptom, who had no indications for coronary angiography. Consequently the studies including a broader spectrum of patients were more representative. In these studies (137-141) patients with major factors for the development of endothelial dysfunction (arterial hypertension, hypercholesterolemia, diabetes, smoking) were excluded. In the above cited, invasive studies, no exclusion of such patients caused that the observed reduction of EDV could be in part induced by the above mentioned secondary factors predisposing to endothelial dysfunction. In contrast, personal studies were carried out in a selected group of patients, in whom impaired EDV was caused most probably by the primary factor i.e. specific massive thickening of the intima-media layer in the vascular wall, which narrows small transmural arteries and arterioles (116;176). It was proved that the severity of luminal stenosis in resistant vessels was inversely correlated with the degree of reduced coronary flow reserve tested by dipyridamole or adenosine (102;162). As for the mechanism of impaired EDV it seems that massive thickening of the intima-media layer may significantly impair NO diffusion to smooth muscle cells in the vascular wall. On the other hand the generation of NO may also be impaired, as it has been demonstrated that marked degenerative changes occur in endothelial cells in the microcirculation (170;173). In personal studies (137-139;141) the vasomotor response of resistant microvessels was evaluated during stress tests to study mainly EDV. Cold pressor test was found to induce pathological vasoconstriction, even in some asymptomatic and mildly symptomatic patients with hypertrophic cardiomyopathy. This finding may correspond to silent myocardial ischemia detected in some asymptomatic patients during exercise stress test combined with scintigraphy (178). Various stimuli were used [in our study cold pressor test, whereas exercise testing in the study by Udelson et al. (178)], however vasomotor response to both stimuli was highly correlated (r=0,92) in patients with endothelial dysfunction (47). As regards the functional consequence of myocardial ischemia, we (143) demonstrated that cold pressor test in untreated asymptomatic patients impaired early left ventricular filling, which is a result of deteriorated myocardial relaxation. Relaxation is an energy-dependent process, which is very sensitive to ischemia. For this reason deteriorated relaxation is an early manifestation of myocardial ischemia, preceding the subsequent stages of the ischemic cascade (Figure 3-4.). Changes in the ischemic cascade develop gradually during metabolic stress test (augmenting myocardial oxygen consumption) because they are interrelated with the increasing double product (that is heart rate multiplied by systolic blood pressure) along with escalating stress. It is worth emphasizing that even a small increase in the double product at early stage of stress test induces disturbances of myocardial perfusion, which are the first manifestations of the ischemic cascade (see also section 5.4).

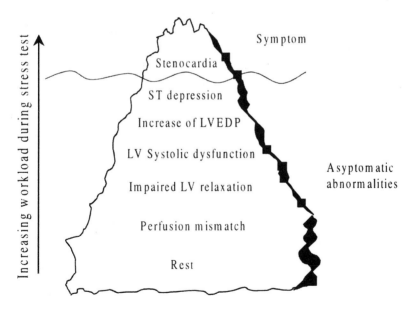

Figure 3-4. The ischemic cascade (displayed as a pyramid-shaped iceberg) developing with increasing workload during metabolic stress test. Anginal pain is a "delayed" symptom in relation to silently progressing abnormalities, which form a larger asymptomatic portion of the iceberg. LVEDP- left ventricular end diastolic pressure

In another personal study (141), using handgrip with moderate force of squeezing [45% of maximal force], it was demonstrated that vasodilator capacity in symptomatic patients with hypertrophic cardiomyopathy was reduced as compared with healthy volunteers. In the most recent study (137), rapid pacing to test EDV induced lesser vasodilator response in patients with hypertrophic cardiomyopathy than in the controls. In all cited studies the beneficial effect of verapamil on coronary vasomotor response to cold pressor test, handgrip and pacing was reported.

3.2   Assessment of epicardial coronary artery stenosis

3.2.1   Functional assessment of stenosis

Two methods are used to functionally assess the severity of coronary stenosis:
–   direct assessment of stenosis by measurement of trans-stenotic pressure gradient
–   coronary flow reserve measured distally to stenosis

An improvement of the first method may be the measurement of trans-stenotic gradient after the administration of a vasodilator. The values obtained during maximal vasodilatation, together with the mean arterial (systemic) pressure (MAP) allow us to calculate coronary fractional flow reserve (FFR) similar as in invasive studies (see section 2.3.1).

The modified formula for echocardiographic calculations will be as follows:

$$FFR = \frac{MAP - \text{mean trans-stenotic gradient}}{MAP}$$

Figure 3.5. and 3.6. are an illustration of echocardiographic measurements of trans-stenotic pressure gradient and FFR.

Figure 3-5. Trans-stenotic pressure gradient measured by transthoracic Doppler echocardiography in patients with significant stenosis in proximal segment of LAD at coronary angiogram. Spectral Doppler tracings of coronary flow velocity was recorded at site of stenosis: [A] pre-PTCA baseline (max. gradient 20,4 mmHg and calculated mean gradient 7,3 mmHg); [B] pre-PTCA peak adenosine (max. gradient 61,3 mmHg and calculated mean gradient 37,4 mmHg); [C] post-PTCA baseline (max. gradient 2,6 mmHg and calculated mean gradient 0,80 mmHg); [D] post-PTCA peak adenosine (max. gradient 14,3 mmHg and calculated mean gradient 4,5 mmHg).

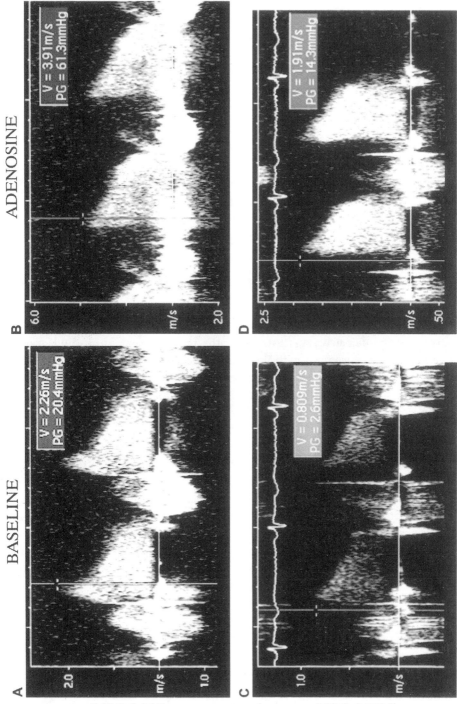

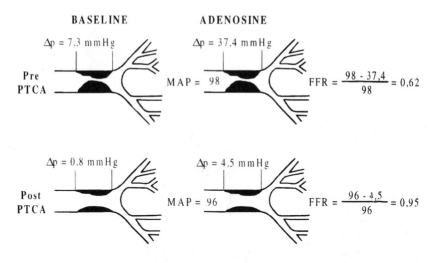

Figure 3-6. Supplementary scheme to previous figure 3-5. Mean value of trans-stenotic pressure gradient (ΔP) and calculated FFR are presented. MAP - mean arterial (systemic) pressure.

Using the measurements obtained only at rest, the first method may be developed in such a way as to replace the measurement of absolute trans-stenotic pressure gradient with the ratio of stenotic to pre-stenotic coronary blood flow velocity (78;158). The second method indirectly assesses the degree of stenosis through the measurement of coronary flow reserve distally to the stenosis (20;22;79;105;146) and is especially useful, if for technical reasons we cannot directly visualize the stenotic site. Importantly, coronary flow reserve can be underestimated, if measured erroneously at the stenosis site, which features relatively high baseline velocity (see figure 3-5A.). Thus, coronary blood flow velocity >0,50 m/s according to Caiati et al. (20-22) and >2m/s according to Krzanowski et al. (103) possibly indicates acceleration at stenosis site. To confirm stenosis, a second Doppler sampling (reference value) must be obtained in a different portion of the artery (20-22;103). According to Krzanowski et al. (103) a local velocity increase with at least doubled maximal velocity within the stenosis as compared with the velocity within the adjacent segment of the artery is regarded as a sign of hemodynamically significant stenosis.

3.2.2   Coronary flow reserve in coronary artery disease

Practically coronary flow reserve for functional assessment of the degree of stenosis may be measured in the following clinical settings:
–   Functional assessment of intermediate (borderline) stenosis (40%-70%)
–   Detection of critical stenosis

- Monitoring of restenosis after PTCA
- Assessment of the PTCA effect on coronary flow reserve
- Measurement of postinfarction coronary flow reserve
- Assessment of coronary graft patency.

3.2.2.1   Functional assessment of intermediate (borderline) stenosis

Coronary angiography provides a limited insight into the physiological significance of coronary stenosis. Understanding the functional impact of stenosis is important for clinical decision making (for example to refer or defer patients with intermediate stenosis to PTCA). The treatment of patients with moderate stenoses is challenging, and coronary flow reserve measured distally to stenosis may be helpful to determine the hemodynamic significance of stenosis. Studies using transthoracic Doppler echocardiography demonstrated that in intermediate stenosis coronary flow reserve ranged widely from 1,5 to 3,5 (19;20;22;42;79;105). The measurement of coronary flow reserve by transthoracic Doppler echocardiography provides data equivalent to those obtained by thallium-201 scintigraphy for physiologic estimation of the severity of LAD stenosis. Importantly, coronary flow reserve < 2,0 is associated with stress-induced ischemia (19;42). In patients with intermediate stenosis but an adequate coronary flow reserve value, PTCA can be safely deferred. For this reason it has been proposed that noninvasive measurement of coronary flow reserve < 2,0 may be useful when deciding about referring to PTCA (19;20;22;42)

3.2.2.2   Detection of critical stenosis

Studies by Gould et al. (59;60) and Klocke (98) demonstrated that stenosis 88% to 93% causes complete exhaustion of coronary flow reserve (see Fig. 2-1., section 2.2.). Using transthoracic Doppler echocardiography it is possible to detect severe LAD stenosis >90%. Coronary flow reserve <1,0; suggesting coronary flow steal phenomenon may be a predictor of critical coronary stenosis in LAD (33;146). This type of coronary flow steal is defined as vertical i.e. resulting from competition for flow supply between stenosed LAD and unstenosed Cx. Subsequently, at maximal coronary vasodilatation, coronary flow decreases in the vascular region supplied by the stenotic artery in favor of the area supplied by the normal artery.

3.2.2.3   Monitoring of restenosis after PTCA

Serial coronary flow reserve examinations during follow-up after PTCA are feasible to monitor restenosis (111;130;131;179). Decreased coronary flow reserve < 2,0 during follow-up was proposed as a sensitive and specific predictor of restenosis (130;179). This method may be complementary to exercise test, or may be its substitute if patients are unable to perform adequate exercise test. In clinical practice a significant portion of patients is not able to exercise because of the following diseases: neurological, respiratory, peripheral vascular (frequently coincident with coronary artery disease) or orthopedic. Additionally, echocardiographic measurement of coronary flow reserve using pharmacological vasodilators is useful in patients with deviation in ST-T segment at baseline ECG (by left bundle branch block, WPW preexcitation syndrome) or in patients who could not reach the target heart rate (85% of maximal predicted heart rate). The latter problem concerns especially elderly patients or patients taking cardiovascular drugs that blunt the heart rate response to exercise (beta-blocker, verapamil) .

Instead of coronary flow reserve measurements distally to stenosis another method has been developed to detect restenosis after PTCA. In some patients direct imaging of the stenosis/restenosis site in LAD is possible if a sufficiently long portion of LAD is visible (158). The (re)-stenotic site is identified as localized color aliasing corresponding to local flow acceleration with turbulence. It is proposed to quantify the severity of restenosis by measuring the increase of coronary blood flow velocity (ratio of stenotic to pre-stenotic velocities) (78). It has been found that the 3-fold increase in stenotic velocity with 100% sensitivity and 100% specificity identifies 50% stenosis by coronary angiography (158). In another study (78) the reverse ratio (pre-stenotic/stenotic velocity) was calculated and the value <0,45 (i.e. >2,22 upon recalculation as the preceding parameter), with 86% sensitivity and 93% specificity predicted restenosis after PTCA.   It should be remembered that these first studies were carried out in relatively small groups of patients.

3.2.2.4   Assessment of PTCA effect on coronary flow reserve

It is desirable to measure coronary flow reserve serially early after PTCA and further days, when coronary flow reserve may fall paradoxically or there is no expected rise of coronary flow reserve (131;146;182;185). A surprisingly high rate of impaired coronary flow reserve immediately after PTCA or stenting, even in the absence of any residual angiographic stenosis was observed as a persistent or transient phenomenon (182;185). This paradoxical phenomenon may derive from:

– Limited increase of maximal hyperemic coronary flow due to periprocedural microvascular damage in distal vascular bed (for details see section 2.3.2)
– Reactive hyperemia, where high post-PTCA baseline flow velocity reduces coronary flow reserve.

The microvascular injury may be responsible for anginal pain after PTCA and perfusion defects in scintigraphy (185). Invasive measurement of coronary flow reserve (immediately after PTCA) may be unreliable because it is obtained after multiple balloon inflations, injection of contrast agent and administration of vasoactive drugs that may produce vasomotor instability. For these reasons, the measurement of coronary flow reserve should be delayed several days after PTCA. At this time, the influence of PTCA-related pharmacological, metabolic, humoral or myogenic factors affecting coronary flow autoregulation is negligible, possibly explaining the lower rate of postprocedural impaired coronary flow reserve in a recent study using transthoracic Doppler echocardiography (146). On the other hand no significant increase in coronary flow reserve several days after the procedure as a result of microvascular damage may occur even in patients undergoing PTCA followed by stent implantation. Early reocclusion of the coronary artery is another complication after PTCA detectable by transthoracic Doppler echocardiography (131).

3.2.2.5 Postinfarction coronary flow reserve assessment

There are several recent reports concerning the value of coronary flow reserve measured transthoracically after reperfused acute anterior myocardial infarct (32;38;180). The first study (32) examined the relationship between coronary flow reserve and no-reflow phenomenon (a marker of microvascular damage). Preserved coronary flow reserve (the cutoff value >2,5) 48 hours after the infarction was associated with smaller microvascular no-reflow extent. Additionally, measurement of coronary flow reserve predicts myocardial viability and functional recovery assessed by global wall motion score index during dobutamine stress echocardiography. In the second study (180) the decreased coronary flow reserve <1,5 was identified to predict an increase in left ventricular volume (remodeling) after reperfused myocardial infarct. A significant negative correlation was found between coronary flow reserve and progression of left ventricular dilatation at 6-month follow-up. In the third study (38) it was shown that preconditioning due to preinfarction angina had a protective role on microvascular function as demonstrated by coronary flow reserve preservation (>2,5) after myocardial infarct.

3.2.2.6 Assessment of coronary graft patency

Transthoracic echocardiography may also be employed to assess the left internal mammary artery used as a bypass to the LAD. The superficial course of the internal mammary artery allows for the detection of flow signal in a high proportion of cases (54). Additionally, the site of bypass and LAD anastomosis is possible to image in around 80% of cases. In a satisfactory proportion of patients with venous bypass it is also possible to detect coronary blood flow in the bypass and visualize the anastomotic site with

LAD (54). De Simone et al. (43) proposed two parameters to evaluate the efficacy of the bypass graft: the ratio of maximal flow velocity at diastole to maximal flow velocity at systole (normal value 1,79±0,47; values below 1,0 imply significant stenosis). The sensitivity and specificity of this index was estimated to be 100% and 58%, respectively. Another parameter is the evaluation of coronary flow reserve tested by dipyridamole, which in normal bypasses was 1,8±0,4, whereas in stenotic bypasses it was practically abolished, because coronary flow reserve was around 1,0. In the most recent and largest study (36) the identification rate for mammary artery grafts was 100%, for saphenous vein grafts to LAD 91%, for vein grafts to right coronary artery 96% and for vein grafts to circumflex artery 90%. Coronary flow reserve<1,9 had 100% sensitivity, 98% specificity for mammary artery graft stenosis. Coronary flow reserve<1,6 had 91% sensitivity, 87% specificity for significant vein graft stenosis.

3.2.3   Abnormalities in resting pattern of coronary flow velocity

Analysis of the pattern of resting coronary flow velocity in the distal LAD is applicable to detect occluded coronary artery (73;134). The retrograde diastolic flow shown both in color-Doppler flow mapping as well as spectral Doppler is a marker of artery occlusion. In a large study group (73) the specificity of reverse diastolic flow for occlusion detection was 100%. However, the sensitivity was lower (i.e. 71,4%), because in some patients collateral vessels supplied the LAD proximally to its distal portion and therefore normal forward diastolic flow was imaged in distal LAD. In these circumstances the retrograde intramyocardial collateral flow signal running through ventricular septum toward the LAD is possible to image (192). The detection of occluded distal portion of RCA is also possible (134).

Severe coronary stenosis (>85%) is detectable based upon the value of resting coronary flow velocity distally to stenosis, on condition that spectral Doppler tracings are recordable both at diastole and systole. The reduced peak diastolic-to-systolic velocity ratio may indicate severe LAD stenosis i.e. 1,3±0,4 versus 1,9±0,5 in patients without significant stenosis p<0,0001 (68). For percent diameter stenosis > 85%, the best cut-off point was 1,6 (sensitivity 77%, specificity 77,9%). What was important for accurate measurements, the authors excluded patients with several factors influencing the systolic-diastolic velocity ratio such as: left ventricular hypertrophy, systemic hypertension and myocardial infarction.

Chapter 4

NONINVASIVE METHODS FOR EVALUATION OF CORONARY FLOW RESERVE - METHODOLOGICAL CONSIDERATIONS

Introduction

Noninvasive techniques for evaluation of myocardial blood supply can be divided into two subgroups. The first subgroup includes Doppler echocardiography, which measures the local blood flow velocity in one of the major coronary arteries supplying a given myocardial region. Color and spectral Doppler techniques are used in transthoracic and transesophageal echocardiography. An accepted simplification of Doppler measurement of coronary blood flow is a measurement not of the volumetric, absolute coronary flow, but only its component i.e. the velocity. The relationship between these two parameters is expressed in the following formula:

Volumetric coronary flow=coronary flow velocity × vessel cross-sectional area

Another approach is to determine perfusion directly in a given myocardial region. The tools we can use are myocardial contrast echocardiography, positron emission tomography (PET), magnetic resonance imaging and ultra-fast computer tomography. PET has an established diagnostic role (it is considered as gold standard), whereas the application of the remaining techniques to quantitatively assess perfusion is just now developing. In an attempt to reproduce the methodology of PET study regional coronary perfusion is quantified by means of myocardial contrast echocardiography. Myocardial contrast echocardiography is used to evaluate blood volume in a given myocardial region after contrast enhancement of the blood signal. At present myocardial contrast echocardiography is based upon one of the four techniques: Harmonic Power Doppler, Harmonic B-mode, Pulse Inversion Imaging, Power Pulse Inversion (11). These techniques are excellently described in a book by Becher and Burns (11) available in the electronic version at *http://www.swchsc.on.ca/EchoHandbook/* .

According to experts (11) comparing the capacity of echocardiographic methods in patients with technically difficult conditions for ultrasonographic examination, coronary flow reserve measured by Doppler technique is feasible fairly frequently when perfusion assessment using echocardiographic contrast agents is not adequate.

4.1   Transthoracic Doppler Echocardiography

The potential of transthoracic Doppler echocardiography for evaluation of local blood flow in the coronary vessel is related to the quality of the equipment and experience of the operator. The feasibility of the imaging increases when echocardiographic contrast agents are used. Table 4-1. summarizes the advantages and disadvantages of Doppler technique.

Table 4-1. Advantages and limitations of transthoracic Doppler echocardiography

Advantages
• Noninvasiveness: study can be serially repeated and any study group can be composed (the only limitation are poor technical conditions for ultrasonographic examination)
• Continuous monitoring of coronary flow velocity: allows for comparison of coronary flow velocity relative to the simultaneously measured double product
• Wider availability and lesser costs as compared with intracoronary Doppler and PET

Limitations
• Only regional flow velocity, mainly in the LAD is measured (lower feasibility of flow imaging in Cx and RCA)
• Difficulties in recording the systolic component of coronary flow
• Difficult measurement of volumetric (absolute) coronary flow
• Limitations relating to theta angle (the angle between the Doppler beam and the direction of blood flow in coronary artery)
• High-end ultrasound equipment required
• High experience of the sonographer required

4.1.1   Advantages of the method:

4.1.1.1   Noninvasive measurements

The measurement of coronary blood flow velocity using transthoracic Doppler echocardiography is noninvasive. Therefore, the measurement is unstressed and absolutely safe for the patients. This comfortable examination provides a possibility of repeating the study for a number of times, which in turn allows for evaluation of various stressors and effects of different pharmacological treatment influencing coronary blood flow in a given patient (137-141). An additional advantage is a possibility to examine asymptomatic patients or those with exertion dyspnea and easy fatigability but without anginal pain (ineligible for invasive studies).

Noninvasive measurements of coronary blood flow velocity permit us to select a truly normal, well-defined control group. In personal studies (137;139-141) the control group had been precisely selected out of healthy volunteers without cardiovascular complaints. An additional entry criterion was a lack of major factors predisposing to endothelial dysfunction (hypertension, smoking, diabetes mellitus, hypercholesterolemia). In many previous invasive studies the controls had not been selected in such a precise manner, which was the shortcoming that could have been eliminated. For ethical reasons it was necessary to select patients with chest pain (and not asymptomatic subjects who would be ideal candidates) as an indication to invasive coronary angiography with complementary measurements of coronary blood flow. This way of defining the controls in invasive studies had already been criticized (115). In previous invasive studies, patients with slow coronary blood flow generally were not excluded from the control group. Consequently patients with syndrome X, characterized by increased resistance in coronary microcirculation could have been included among the controls. In such patients, despite angiographically normal epicardial coronary artery, coronary flow reserve may be markedly limited, even to the level of 1,37 (21).

4.1.1.2 Benefits from continuous monitoring of coronary blood flow velocity during stress test

An additional advantage of Doppler echocardiography is a possibility of simultaneous measurement of coronary flow velocity and double product, which allows for comparison of coronary flow velocity changes in relation to double product increments during stress test. In a metabolic stress test (cold pressor test, handgrip exercise, rapid pacing), such coronary flow normalization to myocardial oxygen demand is indispensable for correct interpretation of the results, because the mechanism of stress testing is a provocation of increased myocardial oxygen consumption, in response to which coronary blood supply should appropriately increase in normal coronary circulation (see section 5.4.1.).

4.1.2   Limitations of the method

4.1.2.1   Feasibility of coronary artery imaging

A major limitation of the technique is impossibility to image coronary blood flow, however only in a minority of study patients. The capacity of coronary flow recording depends mainly on the location of the searched artery. The blood flow velocity is most successfully measured in the LAD, whose middle and distal portion is most accessible and easy to visualize, whereas measurements of blood flow in Cx or RCA are less frequently obtained (103). Initially LAD was imaged only in its middle and distal segments, which lie in the anterior ventricular groove close to the anterior chest wall (see figure 3-1. in chapter 3). With progress in technology and operators' experience deeper lying coronary arteries or their portions have been gradually penetrated. Consequently in some patients it is possible to visualize proximal segments of LAD as well as some segments of Cx, RCA and its branch right posterior descending coronary artery. The method to visualize the right posterior descending branch differs from the technique to image LAD flow. LAD blood flow can be assessed by using high frequency transducers due to proximity of this artery to the chest wall. However this technique is not suitable for imaging peripheral RCA flow because of the greater distance between the transducer and the basal inferior cardiac wall. Therefore a lower frequency transducer is required. In some patients, the coronary circulation is "left dominant" which means that the territories of posterior descending and the posterolateral left ventricular branch are supplied by the Cx. In these cases the diameter of posterior descending branch might be too small to acquire an accurate Doppler flow profile. According to Voci et al. (189) coronary flow reserve is measurable in posterior descending branch arising from RCA in 75% of study patients and arising from Cx in 50% of study patients. Recording an accurate Doppler signal is often hampered by respiratory excursion (enhanced by adenosine). This problem can be partially resolved by obtaining Doppler signals in apnea or by using specific A_{2A} adenosine receptor agonists provoking little or no hyperpnea (see section 5.1.1.)

In pioneer studies on coronary flow velocity using transthoracic echocardiography (without guidance of color Doppler flow mapping), the feasibility of coronary flow imaging was low i.e. 33% (152) and 50% (53). Progress in imaging was associated with using new generation equipment and approach of combining guided color Doppler flow mapping with spectral Doppler (39;79;91;103;140;190). In unselected patients consecutively entering these studies, the feasibility of coronary flow imaging in LAD (without echocardiographic contrast agents) was 34-96%

(39;79;91;103;137-141;190) (table 4-2.). In studies with a contrast-enhancing agent (Levovist) combined with second harmonic Doppler imaging (20-22), coronary flow velocity in the distal or mid portion of the LAD may be measured almost in all patients (Table 4-2.).

Table 4-2. Comparative feasibility of coronary flow imaging in LAD by transthoracic Doppler echocardiography.

Patients	Systolic CBF	Diastolic CBF	References
	Without contrast agents		
CAD	17%	94%	(79)
CAD, VHD, DCM	34% (a)	34% (a)	(91)
CP, normal LAD	56% (a)	56% (a)	(40)
HCM	71% (a)	71% (a)	(39)
CAD, VHD, HT	<76% (b)	76%	(190)
CAD	96%	96%	(146)
CAD	83%	87%	(68)
HCM	71%	71%	(138)
Healthy volunteers HCM	81% 71%	81% 81%	(140)
Healthy volunteers HCM	Nst Nst	75% 80%	(139)
Healthy volunteers HCM	Nst Nst	83% 87%	(141)
	With contrast agents		
CAD, syndrome X	67%	88-100%	(22)
CAD, CP	71%	98%	(20)
Not stated	100%	100%	(21)
a- studies in patients with adequate imaging both of systolic and diastolic coronary blood flow velocity, b- no exact data (investigators stated only that systolic coronary blood flow was not recorded in all patients with diastolic coronary blood flow), Nst- not studied (details in the text), CBF- coronary blood flow , CAD- coronary artery disease, VHD-valvular heart disease, DCM- dilated cardiomyopathy, HCM- hypertrophic cardiomyopathy, CP- chest pain, HT- hypertension			

In assessment of coronary flow in LAD, the learning curve effect was seen in most centers in which contrast agents were not used. In studies by

Shapiro and coworkers, which were initiated in the beginning of the 90s, the capacity of detecting coronary flow increased from 34% to 77% (39;40;71;91). Voci and coworkers were able to increase the capacity of coronary blood flow imaging from 76% (190) to 96% (146). This result is fully comparable with the results of studies using contrast agents. In personal studies the capacity of detection increased with time and experience from 71% to 87% (138-140). Only Hozumi et al. (79) achieved a very high feasibility of coronary flow imaging already in their first study, i.e. 94%.

High quality images are more difficult to obtain in patients with obesity and emphysema (91), whereas myocardial hypertrophy is a facilitating factor because hypertrophy induces a compensatory increase in the vessel caliber (39;91;96).

4.1.2.2   Feasibility of recording maximal coronary blood flow velocity at peak stress

While testing coronary flow reserve using pharmacological stimuli it was not possible to successfully image the coronary blood flow velocity at peak stress in all patients in whom resting (baseline) coronary flow was recorded. The excellent feasibility of coronary flow reserve measurement using dipyridamole was reported in a study by Rigo et al. (151). The feasibility was 93% in first 100 patients and rose to 98% in a further series of 139 patients. In a larger group of patients (957 patients), the feasibility of coronary flow reserve was 92% for dipyridamole, 90% for adenosine and 71% for dobutamine (111). It is noteworthy that pharmacological stressing with dobutamine (increasing myocardial oxygen demand) is most frequently an obstacle to record high-quality Doppler spectrum of coronary blood flow velocity at peak stress. In personal studies (137-139;141) using physiological stimuli to increase myocardial oxygen demand, coronary flow velocity at peak stress was successfully obtained in all patients. The higher feasibility in these studies may result from a lower level of workload during stress testing.

4.1.2.3   Systolic component of coronary blood flow velocity

In studies without contrast agents marked variation in the feasibility of coronary flow velocity measurement between investigators may result from a methodologically different approach to evaluate the biphasic pattern of systolic-diastolic coronary flow. Some investigators accepted a spectral Doppler recording as adequate only when both systolic and diastolic components of coronary flow velocity were detected (Table 4-2.), whereas according to other investigators the recording of only the diastolic component was sufficient for analysis (Table 4-2.). The latter, more liberal approach may be accounted for by a marked dominance of diastolic over systolic coronary blood flow. With this simplified manner of detection more measurements have been accepted as adequate. An example of marked variation is provided by a study by Hozumi et al. (79), who recorded diastolic coronary flow in 94% of patients, and systolic only in 17%. In contrast, a high success rate (83%) to detect systolic coronary blood flow was reported in an impressively large study by Higashi et al. (68). According to the authors, the use of long sampling volume (5 mm) provides an opportunity to maintain adequate sampling of the pulsed Doppler signal of the LAD flow throughout the cardiac cycle despite cyclic cardiac motion.

In patients with hypertrophic cardiomyopathy, when recording the spectrum of systolic coronary flow additional obstacles may be encountered. From precise invasive studies (1;104) we know that in patients with hypertrophic cardiomyopathy the systolic coronary flow velocity is decreased, and in some patients coronary flow may cease or become retrograde. The retrograde flow is usually slow (1). Low blood flow velocity in a coronary vessel is difficult to record. It may be eliminated by high-pass filters or may be superimposed by artifacts – cardiac wall motion, which is characterized by similar slow velocities. Summing up, decreased coronary flow velocity to several cm/s (irrespective of the flow direction) may be difficult to record by Doppler echocardiography.

Another obstacle in evaluating systolic coronary blood flow is related to stress testing, which may increase contractility of left ventricular walls. In these circumstances the range of arterial motion increases, being totally or partially displaced outside the Doppler beam at systole. In this situation the conditions for recording systolic coronary blood flow deteriorate (174).

4.1.2.4 Coronary flow velocity as a substitute for volumetric coronary blood flow

Volumetric coronary flow is a product of coronary flow velocity and vessel cross-sectional area. A limitation of transthoracic echocardiography is that it measures accurately flow velocity, whereas the measurement of small changes in vessel caliber may be imprecise in some patients. In previous studies (40;70) the measurement of LAD diameter was possible only in 44%-63% of patients. Therefore in most studies, only the changes in coronary flow velocity were evaluated during stress testing. The results are reliable and representative, because resistant vessels of the microcirculation are mainly responsible for changes in coronary blood flow, whereas epicardial arteries (as conductance vessels) contribute in a minor degree to coronary flow regulation (see table 1-1. and section 1.2.). This theory is confirmed by a previously found strong correlation between increments in coronary blood flow velocity and absolute (volumetric) coronary blood flow increase, induced by stimuli activating EDV or EIDV (21;121;149;150;157;195). The strongest correlation was r=0,94 (p<0,0001), which indicates a practically ideal concordance between these two methods (157). The measurement of coronary flow velocity was used as a valuable substitute for absolute coronary blood flow, to calculate coronary flow reserve in large trials such as DEBATE (144;163;164) DESTINI (45) and FROST (49), which show that this simplification was accepted even in invasive studies, where the vessel caliber may be measured precisely.

4.1.2.5   Limitations of Doppler method and pitfalls in the assessment of coronary flow

Limitations of Doppler technique, which may underestimate of real coronary flow velocity, include problems associated with the achievement of theta angle as minimal as possible. Theta angle is the angle between Doppler beam and the direction of blood flow in coronary artery and cannot exceed 45 degrees (precise manual correction is needed if angle is between 20-45 degree). A desirable value of theta angle is <30 degree. However, the shortcomings of an undesirably large theta angle become unimportant, if we compare blood velocity measured continuously in the same site of the vessel before and during stress test. The expression of changes in blood velocity as the ratio of flow velocity during stress testing and velocity at baseline makes the result independent of theta angle, whose value must be constant during stress test. The basic assumptions of the method is that the theta angle is kept constant throughout the examination. One way to reach this goal is to maintain the same view throughout examination with no interruption of imaging.

Several pitfalls should be considered when coronary blood flow is assessed using transthoracic echocardiography. These include fluid in pericardial space, extracardiac thoracic arteries and thoracic veins. Flow in these structures can be distinguished from the characteristic coronary blood flow signal by specific Doppler criteria. Pulsed wave Doppler recording of pericardial fluid flow shows rapid increase in flow velocity during early systole caused by the cardiac contraction. Extracardiac thoracic artery shows predominant systolic flow. Additionally, this artery can be recognized by its lack of cardiac motion.

Using the echocardiographic contrast agents is associated with problem of microbubbles noise. Microbubbles noise appearing as a series of spikes in the Doppler spectrum, represents disruption of microbubbles by ultrasound pressure as they pass through the Doppler beam. These spikes in the spectrum hamper a precise delineation of the spectral Doppler tracing. This noise can be partially avoided by reducing transmit power (mechanical index).

4.2   Transesophageal Doppler echocardiography

Transesophageal echocardiography is a semi-invasive method allowing us to image only the left main coronary artery and proximal segments of LAD, Cx, RCA, with the latter two arteries being less visible (88-90). Stenosis in proximal segments of these arteries may be identified using the following techniques:
- spectral Doppler,
- color Doppler,
- imaging with 3-dimensional reconstruction.

The first two methods are based upon evaluation of coronary blood flow, the third method upon morphological analysis of the artery. Coronary flow reserve can be measured only from coronary flow velocity obtained by spectral Doppler.

4.2.1   Feasibility of spectral Doppler

Analysis of coronary flow velocity by spectral Doppler is characterized by the following limitations: theta angle allows for a reliable measurement of flow velocity more frequently in LAD than Cx and RCA. According to Kasprzak et al. (88-90) who studied a large group of 210 patients, the feasibility of coronary flow velocity measurement was 88% (left main coronary artery), 85% (LAD), 58% (Cx) and 65% (RCA).

Unfortunately coronary flow reserve measured in the proximal LAD is characterized by certain shortcomings, which limit the use of transesophageal Doppler echocardiography. Coronary flow reserve measured only in the proximal LAD is reliable for evaluation of the microcirculation only on condition that there is no stenosis in the distal LAD and its all important branches are normal (21). In these circumstances coronary flow reserve dependent on the microcirculation is tested precisely [e.g. in patients with syndrome X, arterial hypertension, hypertrophic cardiomyopathy (101;122;136)]. In case of stenosis distally to the measurement site, coronary flow reserve is overestimated in relation to true post-stenotic value (21), (see also introduction in chapter 3 and figure 3-3., which explains this problem). When evaluating stenosis directly in the proximal vessel, coronary flow velocity measured even at rest may be valuable. The accelerated flow velocity is a direct indicator of stenosis. Kasprzak et al. (88;89) proposed cut-off values for coronary flow velocity to distinguish between normal and stenosed vessels.

**4.2.2   Assessment of coronary blood flow by color Doppler –
             identification of stenotic site**

Color Doppler is more feasible than spectral Doppler in direct assessment of stenosis in proximal coronary arteries. Accordingly, color Doppler images blood flow in the left main coronary artery (in 99,5% of patients), in LAD (in 96,7% of patients), in Cx (in 98,6% of patients), and RCA (in 95,2% of patients) (88). In order to detect stenosis it is helpful to identify two pathological features of blood flow: turbulence and aliasing. These two pathological phenomena are sensitive and specific predictors for angiographically documented stenosis, however only in the left main artery and proximal LAD (88). In contrast, the sensitivity of Color Doppler to identify stenosis in Cx and RCA is lower, with the specificity being the same (88).

4.2.3   Morphological imaging of the coronary artery

Three-dimensional reconstruction is an important progress in imaging the morphology of coronary vessels by transesophageal echocardiography (196). This innovation allows for imaging proximal LAD in 100%, Cx in 98% and RCA in 72%. The recorded images are used to evaluate stenosis in the visualized arterial segments. Comparison between echocardiographic 3-dimensional reconstruction and coronary angiography in semiquantitative estimation of coronary stenosis resulted in a complete agreement in 83% of the segments. The sensitivity and specificity of this echocardiographic method in detecting stenosis >50% were 84% and 97% respectively.

**4.2.4   Limitations of transesophageal echocardiography in coronary
             blood flow imaging**

Transesophageal echocardiography is inconvenient method for serial measurements of coronary flow velocity, as it is semi-invasive, and it is not well tolerated by patients, especially when the study is combined with dipyridamole administration. An additional disadvantage is a lack of verbal contact with the patient during provocative testing of coronary flow reserve. Consequently the patient is not able to report "on-line" any possible complaints (for instance the development of stenocardia as a result of stressing). Furthermore baseline measurements of coronary blood flow cannot be regarded as values characteristic of resting conditions, because transducer insertion is a stressful situation making patient's discomfort, which is reflected in an elevated value (up to 9000-10000) of double product (149). In contrast in PET or during transthoracic echocardiography baseline double product is 7000-8000 on average (137;140;141;149;157). Kasprzak et al. (89;90) in their study confirm that increased coronary flow velocity is correlated with higher heart rate, a component of double product.

An attempt to eliminate stress associated with the examination by means of intravenous sedative agents may induce systemic blood pressure fall (149). Arterial hypotension significantly alters hemodynamic conditions of the study inducing a decrease in coronary perfusion pressure and may force us to terminate prematurely the study, when the pressure fall is marked (149).

4.3   Positron Emission Tomography

PET is a technique competing with echocardiography. Its advantages include a possibility of measuring absolute coronary blood flow and assessment of blood flow both in a given region of the myocardium or globally. Its disadvantages are quite numerous, as it is a less available tool, it is expensive and exposes the patient to radiation. An additional shortcoming of PET may be a failure of precise, simultaneous measurement of instantaneous values of coronary blood flow and double product. As data acquisition in PET is prolonged, it is not possible to correlate precisely coronary blood flow with double product in case of dynamically changing parameters, for instance at peak exercise and immediately upon exercise cessation. In case of dipyridamole infusion a methodological simplification is to arbitrarily assume that maximal vasodilatation occurs at 8 min after the onset of infusion and data acquisition is focused on this time point (149). This assumption is not necessarily correct, because the second infusion of dipyridamole with continuously monitored coronary blood flow by transesophageal Doppler echocardiography demonstrated that maximal vasodilatation may occur between the 3rd and 12th minute, most frequently outside the arbitrarily assumed time point of 8 min for PET (149). The suggestion that PET measurements of coronary flow reserve after dipyridamole are random in character (and therefore maximal coronary flow is not always captured) is confirmed by a wide scatter of coronary flow reserve measurements by PET defined as normal. The range of normal limits is broad from 2,5 to 5,5 (41;82;110;181;185) (table 2-1., section 2.1.1.). Iida et al. (82) obtained the mean value of coronary flow reserve 3,8±2,1. A considerably high standard deviation confirms the significant scatter of measurements in individual patients. Analyzing the results of this study, it seems that in some healthy volunteers the low value of coronary flow reserve (around 2,5) could have resulted from the possibility that the measurement of coronary blood flow fell outside the moment of maximal vasodilatation.   Additionally the authors suggested that underestimated coronary flow reserve might have derived from a possibility that some volunteers might have taken caffeine-containing foods or drinks before study despite instruction to be fasted.

Summing up, PET cannot measure continuously, consecutive, rapidly occurring dynamic changes in coronary blood flow during stress testing. Doppler echocardiography is free from these limitations, because changes in coronary flow velocity can be monitored continuously.

Chapter 5

STIMULI TESTING CORONARY FLOW RESERVE

Introduction

A wide panel of stimuli can be used to induce changes in coronary blood flow. Generally the stimuli can be divided into those decreasing (NO synthase inhibitors) or increasing coronary blood flow via EDV or EIDV. The former stimuli induce transient endothelial dysfunction in the normal coronary circulation. The latter group of stimuli testing EDV is variable. Generally these stimuli increase coronary blood flow in the normal coronary circulation, whereas in the presence of endothelial dysfunction they may blunt the augmentation of coronary blood flow or even reduce blood flow (see Figure 1-6.). Table 5-1. below summarizes the stimuli affecting coronary blood flow.

Table 5-1. Stimuli testing coronary flow reserve may be classified according to:

I. Mechanisms of action:
- via EDV: cold pressor test, pacing, acetylcholine, substance P, serotonin, bradykinin
- via EIDV: dipyridamole, adenosine, papaverine,

II. Mode of application:
- intracoronary for invasive assessment (acetylcholine, substance P, adenosine),
- intravenous for noninvasive assessment (adenosine, dipyridamole),
- without vasodilator injection (cold pressor test, handgrip exercise),
- rapid atrial pacing:
  - a/ invasive (transvenous stimulation),
  - b/ semi-invasive (transesophageal stimulation) ·
  - c/ noninvasive (stimulation using a previously implanted pacemaker)

III. Effect of action:
- pharmacological vasodilators
- metabolic vasodilators.

Stimuli testing EIDV usually increase . coronary blood flow with two expectations. Decreased hyperemic (post-vasodilator) coronary flow (described as the steal phenomenon) has been observed in patients with critical epicardial stenosis >90% (33;146) and in some patients with hypertrophic cardiomyopathy (172). Nitroglycerine is not listed as it acts selectively on large (epicardial) arteries and therefore it does not affect the microcirculation, which is the principal site of coronary vascular resistance.

5.1 Pharmacological vasodilators testing endothelium-independent vasodilatation

5.1.1 Comparison between adenosine and dipyridamole

In pharmacological tests, EIDV is evaluated mainly using dipyridamole and adenosine, which have replaced the previously used papaverine. The mechanism of action both of adenosine and dipyridamole has been described in section 1.2.3. Table 5-2. contains comparative characteristics of the two vasodilator agents.

Table 5-2. Comparison of pharmacological vasodilators

	Adenosine	Dipyridamole
Route of administration and dosage	Intravenous (i.v.) - 140 µg/kg/min Intracoronarily to LAD (i.c.) – 12-54 µg (bolus)	Intravenous - 0,56-0,84 mg/kg
Duration of action	30 sec	30 min
Time to maximal effect	10 sec i.c. 30-55 sec i.v.	6-16 min
Advantage	Short action, i.v. infusion suitable for noninvasive testing	i.v. infusion suitable for noninvasive testing
Disadvantage	AV conduction delay (including complete heart block), Hyperventilation, hypotension, flushing, headache,	Submaximal vasodilatation, possibility of antidote-resistance prolonged ischemia, prolonged action, hypotension, flushing, headache, hyperventilation
Drug interaction	24-hour abstention from caffeine-containing foods or drinks and 48-hour abstention from slow release theophylline (competitive adenosine receptor antagonists) is required	
Contraindications	Absolute: Active bronchospasm 2nd and 3rd degree atrioventricular block, hypotension Relative: History of spastic (obstructive) airway disease Severe sinus bradycardia or sick sinus syndrome	

Intravenous adenosine is a more expensive vasodilator but superior to dipyridamole. Adenosine rapidly induces vasodilatation, and peak effect is achieved faster. The offset of adenosine action is also rapid. Consequently, the hyperemic part of the study is shorter and associated with prompt reversibility of the side effects, if any, after termination of the infusion with no need for antidote, making adenosine safe and well accepted by the patients (6;22;146;154). The examination using adenosine is less time-consuming. Adenosine infusion may induce specific side effect i.e. transitory (short-lasting) complete heart block. Therefore it is recommended to reduce the dosage of adenosine injected directly to right coronary artery. Another shortcoming of adenosine infused intravenously is induced hyperpnea. Hyperventilation may be disturbing for the patients, however prompt reversibility of this side effect after termination of the adenosine infusion makes this drug safe and acceptable for patients. When assessing coronary flow reserve in the LAD coronary artery, hyperventilation rarely causes degradation of image quality (22). In contrast, coronary flow reserve in the posterior descending coronary artery is measured at a lower success rate as compared with the LAD. According to Voci et al. (189) coronary flow reserve is measurable in the posterior descending coronary artery arising from RCA in 75% of study patients and arising from Cx in 50% of study patients. This lower success rate is partially related to the fact that adenosine-induced hyperventilation interferes with posterior rather than anterior descending imaging. The use of specific A_{2A} adenosine receptor agonists provoking little or no hyperventilation (95) has been tested to overcome this limitation and improve the feasibility of imaging the posterior descending artery.

Problems relating to dipyridamole will be discussed in detail in further sections.

5.1.2   Problems with inducing maximal vasodilatation

The major issue that arises when giving vasodilators is whether maximal vasodilatation has been achieved. In a number of studies on coronary flow reserve dipyridamole was used in a dose of 0,56 mg/kg (infusion over 4 minutes). The induced coronary flow reserve should be regarded as submaximal, because only after 0,84 mg/kg dipyridamole coronary flow reserve was comparable to that achieved after adenosine (109). However, Holdright et al. (75) found out that even a high dose of dipyridamole (0,84 mg/kg) did not increase coronary flow reserve so high as during adenosine infusion.

Studies in humans demonstrated that increasing doses of dipyridamole or adenosine may induce numerous and sometimes serious side effects. Therefore it is not possible to augment the dose of a vasodilator to any level because of the increasing discomfort to the patient and increased risk for the development of serious complications. When using dipyridamole we cannot practically exceed the dose of 1 mg/kg (0,6 mg/kg over five minutes and after five minute interval a further 0,4 mg/kg infused over five minute) (118), at which 67% of study patients reported side effects (chest pain, headache, dizziness, nausea). It is important to remember that severe complications may develop such as pronounced hypotension; prolonged aminophylline-resistant ischemia, and even cardiac arrest (7;16;108;118)

The need to limit the dose of an intravenous vasodilator most probably does not allow for achieving maximal vasodilatation in humans (74). This theory has been confirmed in experimental studies. It was initially assumed that maximal pharmacological vasodilatation is achieved if the infused vasodilator has induced the flow increment equivalent to post-occlusive reactive hyperemia (previously considered as referential maximal flow) (74). However, an experimental study demonstrated that vasodilatation after reactive hyperemia does not define the threshold of maximal increase in coronary flow reserve (17). When an aggressive combination of increasing doses of papaverine and ATP was infused in animals (17) it was found out that the level of coronary flow reserve induced by reactive hyperemia was doubled from 3,8 to 7,8 (the level practically impossible to achieve in humans).

In invasive measurement of coronary flow reserve with intracoronary infusion of adenosine, an incremental dose of adenosine (from 12 to 54 μg for LAD) should be infused to achieve a more reliable value of coronary flow reserve (46). For example, 27% of patients with intermediate coronary stenoses (40-70%) with an initial coronary flow reserve <2,5 (induced by low dose adenosine) increased its value>2,5 with incremental doses of adenosine (46). In patients with mild coronary artery stenosis (<40%), the percent of subjects with increasing value of reserve was higher i.e. 39% (46).

5.1.3   The impact of variable extent of coronary vasculature

Apart from the dose of infused vasodilator an important factor modifying its concentration in the coronary circulation and consequently the magnitude of coronary flow reserve is the extent of coronary vasculature. The extent of coronary vasculature is partially determined by the amount of myocardial mass supplied by the artery. For this reason it is difficult to compare vasodilator effects between various study groups with varying amounts of the myocardium supplied by LAD (24;101). It has been demonstrated that in myocardial hypertrophy (moderate hypertrophy complicating arterial hypertension) higher doses of dipyridamole are required to increase coronary blood flow to a level similar to, although slightly lower than in the controls (101). This problem may be especially pronounced in hypertrophic cardiomyopathy, where septal mass markedly exceeds normal values. In these circumstances pharmacological vasodilatation using maximal, safely applicable doses of dipyridamole may be a submaximal stimulus relative to the increased extent of coronary vasculature within the massively thickened septum. The postulated effect of hypertrophy on coronary flow reserve seems to be confirmed by a strong correlation (r=0,80) between the increasing septal thickness and the decreasing coronary flow reserve induced by dipyridamole (102). A compensatory increase in the dose of dipyridamole is not possible due to enhanced side effects (118).

A similar problem concerns intracoronary infusion of acetylcholine to test EDV. Given the extent of the coronary vasculature distal to LAD varies from patient to patient, it is possible that some patients with the smaller extent of vasculature distal to the infusion catheter, could have achieved higher intracoronary concentration of acetylcholine than those with greater vasculature (24). In extreme conditions, acetylcholine (especially in high dose) may constrict not dilate coronary artery with normal endothelium.

5.1.4   Summary

Summing up, adenosine should replace dipyridamole in pharmacological testing of coronary flow reserve. Dipyridamole has an intrinsic limitation for coronary flow reserve assessment, especially if it is used in a contrast-enhanced echocardiographic study. Since it takes a long time to reach maximal effect, contrast infusion has to be discontinued after a baseline study and a second infusion of contrast has to be started after dipyridamole infusion (22). Adenosine thanks to its rapid action may overcome most of the shortcomings inherent in using dipyridamole (relatively long duration of the study, need for a larger amount of contrast, reimaging coronary flow during hyperemia, need for an antidote to treat side effects).

5.2   Stimuli increasing myocardial oxygen demand

5.2.1   Adrenergic stimulation

In humans, if it is not possible to achieve truly maximal vasodilatation during pharmacological testing and bearing in mind their limitations we may use alternative submaximal stress tests. These are tests increasing myocardial metabolism and oxygen demand, including cold pressor test, handgrip, exercise test, mental test and rapid atrial pacing (23;47;58;128;129;137-139;141;147;153;155;197-200). These tests are more physiological than pharmacological interventions, as cold pressor test, handgrip, exercise test and mental test activate the adrenergic system and provoke an increase in myocardial metabolic demand. In normal response to these stimuli the coronary flow velocity should increase.

The additional advantage of metabolic stress testing is that it is a natural physiologic stress and mimics the stresses of daily living for the patients better than pharmacological vasodilatation, whose mechanism of action is not related to increasing myocardial oxygen demand.

5.2.1.1   Endogenous catecholamine stimulation

Cold pressor test and handgrip may be combined with transthoracic Doppler echocardiography to study the coronary flow velocity, because spectral Doppler recordings during these stress tests is of acceptable quality in most patients (138;139;141). The most valuable, fully physiological stress testing of the cardiovascular system is an exercise test (on condition the patient is able to perform adequate effort). Unfortunately during an intensive exercise (on a treadmill or bicycle) patients' body motion and hyperventilation practically make impossible the recording of high-quality spectral Doppler tracing using transthoracic echocardiography. Another type of stress test, which for technical reasons is difficult to perform in combination with transthoracic echocardiography, is mental stress. During this test the patient is routinely instructed to perform mathematical operations. The results of consecutive memory operations (for instance serial subtraction of the same one-digit number from a three-digit number) are given by the patients immediately. In this moment the recording of Doppler signal is impaired. Another obstacle in the validation of the study is marked variation in the emotional state of the patient during the test originating from individual predisposition to memory mathematical operations. For obvious reasons the exercise test and mental test cannot be performed during transesophageal echocardiography. In these circumstances coronary blood flow can only be measured noninvasively by means of PET.

5.2.1.2   Exogenous catecholamine stimulation

The above-described tests activating the adrenergic system are based upon the increase in endogenous catecholamines. Exogenous catecholamine stimulation may be their counterpart. Dobutamine as an agent for assessment of coronary blood flow increase has been used both in invasive (104;153) and noninvasive studies (171;174). In noninvasive studies (where dobutamine was combined with atropine) the recording of maximal coronary blood flow was possible at higher heart workload in PET (171) than in transthoracic Doppler echocardiography (174). In the latter case when the heart rate exceeds 130 beats per minute during dobutamine infusion the recording of spectral Doppler velocity profiles of the coronary flow becomes technically unsatisfactory (174).

5.2.2 Pacing

The increase in coronary blood flow, although without the adrenergic stimulation, may be also evoked by pacing-induced tachycardia. Personal studies demonstrated that changes in the coronary flow velocity induced by rapid pacing could be evaluated with satisfactory results using transthoracic Doppler echocardiography (137). Pacing was well tolerated and safe. Importantly, Lee et al. (106) demonstrated that rapid atrial pacing as compared with dobutamine caused less side effects (arrhythmia, hypotension or hypertension episodes) and allowed for the achievement of target heart rate, which was not possible in some patients during dobutamine test.

5.2.3 Advantages of metabolic stress test

Advantage of metabolic stress testing in contrast to pharmacological agents (testing EDV) is noninvasive application of the stimulus (there in no need for intracoronary infusion of acetylcholine, serotonin, substance P, bradykinin). This noninvasive approach increases patient's comfort (it is especially important if the patient has to undergo a series of tests). Physiological tests are very well tolerated by the patient, for instance handgrip test, which may be performed practically by anyone and the level of workload is not fixedly forced but tailored to the individual patient's strength. The use of the constant percent of maximal voluntary contraction (45% in our study) (141) allows for validating the test for further comparative studies for instance after treatment. In the remaining tests (cold pressor test, pacing) the unpleasant stimulus may be immediately withdrawn. In personal studies (138;139) during cold pressor test, two patients out of over 40 removed their hands from the ice water thus interrupting the study, prematurely. In contrast, rapid pacing to 120 beats per minute was accepted by all study patients (137).

5.3 Summary

Pharmacological stimuli used intravenously (dipyridamole, adenosine) i.e. those which may be combined with noninvasive measurement of coronary blood flow verify only EIDV. In contrast, assessment of EDV using pharmacological stimuli requires intracoronary administration (acetylcholine, serotonin, substance P, bradykinin), which is associated with invasiveness. Some metabolic stimuli may be applied noninvasively (cold pressor, handgrip, pacing using a previously implanted pacemaker), or semi-invasively (transesophageal pacing). The previously implanted pacemaker was already used in paced echocardiographic stress test to assess myocardial wall motion abnormalities to diagnose coronary artery disease (12).

5.4 Corrected coronary blood flow in metabolic stress test

5.4.1 Coronary blood flow normalized to double product

Metabolic stress testing consists in provoking an increase in myocardial oxygen demand in response to which coronary blood flow should also increase on condition there are no flow-limiting factors (endothelial dysfunction, vasospasm, epicardial stenosis). If the potential for increasing coronary blood flow is limited, imbalance between the increasing oxygen demand and insufficient myocardial supply develops. This myocardial oxygen supply-demand mismatch may be especially enhanced in the absence of the increase or even with the decreased coronary blood flow during stress testing, which was demonstrated in several previous studies (153;156;199;200).

Thus, for correct interpretation of stress-induced changes in coronary flow velocity it is necessary to compare this value with the increase of an index reflecting myocardial oxygen demand. A widely used indicator is double product (rate-pressure product), i.e. heart rate multiplied by systolic blood pressure. The advantage of this parameter is simplicity of measurement, whereas a disadvantage is a lack of adjustment for altered myocardial contractility.

In earlier reports on metabolic stress testing to assess EDV the data were frequently presented as percent change in coronary blood flow and comparison of double product values at baseline and during a given stress test (104;128;135). This way of presenting the results allowed for only approximate comparison of increments in coronary blood flow in relation to double product. A more precise analysis of the proportional increase in coronary blood flow and double product (or pathological disproportion) is a comparison of percent changes in these parameters. However, only several reports on EDV presented this type of results (23;57;198;199). A more perfect solution seems to be an adequate indicator, which was proposed by Rossen et al. (153). This universal index has been expressed as the ratio of:

$$\frac{\% \text{ change in coronary flow velocity}}{\% \text{ change in double product}}$$

To the best of my knowledge there are no proposals as to the normal value of this index for various stress tests. Rossen et al. (153) studied a group of patients with indications to invasive coronary angiography and with risk factors for endothelial dysfunction (hypertension, diabetes mellitus, no data on smoking), (table 5-3.). During pacing, the investigators most frequently recorded the index value ranging from 0 to 1 (based upon individual patient's data in the diagram we may suspect that the mean value for the whole group does not exceed 0,5). Only one patient reached the index value about 1,0 whereas several patients had a negative index, which reflected severe endothelial dysfunction. This result is interpreted as highly abnormal coronary vasoconstriction despite the increasing myocardial metabolic demand. A shortcoming of this study (153) is no control group. When comparing the results of previous studies with cold pressor test and handgrip (Table 5-3.) it seems that in the control group the ratio of mean percent increase in coronary blood flow to double product should be close to 1 or slightly exceeding 1. Unfortunately most reports lack individual data and therefore the comparison of mean values may be imprecise. Personal studies filled this gap by providing the index value for healthy volunteers undergoing cold pressor test, handgrip test and pacing (137;139;141). For cold pressor and handgrip tests the mean index value exceeded 1, whereas for pacing, the index value was close to 1.

Table 5-3. Proportion of changes in coronary blood flow in relation to altered double product

Study group	Test	%CBF /%DP	Reference
Control group	CPT	> 1 [a]	(198)
Endothelial dysfunction in early atherosclerosis		< 1 [a]	
Control group	CPT	> 1 [a]	(199)
Endothelial dysfunction in early atherosclerosis		< 1 [a]	
Control group	CPT	> 1 [a]	(23)
Cigarette smokers		< 1 [a]	
Healthy volunteers	. HG	around 1	(57)
Endothelial dysfunction in diabetic and HT patients	PACE	around 0,5 [a]	(153)
Healthy volunteers	CPT	> 1	(139)
Hypertrophic cardiomyopathy	CPT	< 1	
Healthy volunteers	HG	> 1	(141)
Hypertrophic cardiomyopathy	HG	< 1	
Control group	PACE	around 1	(137)
Hypertrophic cardiomyopathy	PACE	< 1	
CBF- coronary blood flow, DP – double product, a- estimate values (see details in the text), PACE- pacing, CPT- cold pressor test, HG- handgrip, HT-hypertension			

Double product is a reflection of oxygen demand of the whole myocardium. On the other hand the coronary flow velocity has been measured by Doppler echocardiography only in the LAD, which means that the assessment was local. In case of hypertrophic cardiomyopathy, in which interventricular septum hypertrophy is a dominant feature (in all patients in personal studies), analysis of the local flow in the LAD, which supplies the septum, is of key importance.

5.4.2   Calculation of coronary vascular resistance index

Another way of comparing increased coronary blood flow with hemodynamic changes during stress testing is the determination of the percent change in coronary vascular resistance index (4;83;156;199;200) The index is calculated according to the following formula:

$$\text{Resistance index} = \frac{\text{mean aortic pressure}}{\text{coronary flow velocity (or coronary blood flow if available)}}$$

When analyzing EDV using cold pressor test (199;200) resistance in normal coronary vessels decreases, whereas it increases in case of endothelial dysfunction. Using rapid atrial pacing, which is also used to test EDV, coronary vascular resistance index was decreased by 60% in control group (156). Cannon et al. (27) in patients with non-obstructive hypertrophic cardiomyopathy demonstrated that coronary vascular resistance is decreased to a lesser extent than the figure given above, whereas in obstructive hypertrophic cardiomyopathy coronary vascular resistance during pacing may even slightly increase. In personal studies in untreated patients with hypertrophic cardiomyopathy, cold pressor test was found to increase coronary vascular resistance index, which is a pathological response as compared with the controls (138). Handgrip in patients with hypertrophic cardiomyopathy induces a negligible increase in coronary vascular resistance index, whereas in the controls resistance was found to be decreased during handgrip (141). During pacing at heart rate 120 beats per minute, resistance decreased in patients with hypertrophic cardiomyopathy and in the controls, the reduction being significantly larger in the controls (137). The hypertrophic cardiomyopathy group was not homogenous, because it included patients with obstructive and nonobstructive hypertrophic cardiomyopathy.

When testing EIDV coronary vascular resistance decreases both in the controls and in patients with cardiovascular diseases varying in severity (for instance hypertension with or without left ventricular hypertrophy). For this reason the magnitude of the decrease is a measure of pathological response.

The largest reduction is observed in patients with normal coronary vessels (200). The decrease of coronary vascular resistance after vasodilator is gradually blunt in following sequence: hypertensive patients without left ventricular hypertrophy, hypertensive patients with hypertrophy, untreated hypertensive patients with hypertrophy (4).

REFERENCE LIST

1. Akasaka T, Yoshikawa J, Yoshida K et al. Phasic coronary flow characteristics in patients with hypertrophic cardiomyopathy: a study by coronary Doppler catheter. J.Am.Soc.Echocardiogr. 1994;7:9-19.

2. Anderson TJ, Elstein E, Haber H et al. Comparative study of ACE-inhibition, angiotensin II antagonism, and calcium channel blockade on flow-mediated vasodilation in patients with coronary disease (BANFF study). J.Am.Coll.Cardiol. 2000;35:60-66.

3. Anderson TJ, Gerhard MD, Meredith IT et al. Systemic nature of endothelial dysfunction in atherosclerosis. Am.J.Cardiol. 1995;75:71B-74B.

4. Antony I, Nitenberg A, Foult JM et al. Coronary vasodilator reserve in untreated and treated hypertensive patients with and without left ventricular hypertrophy. J.Am.Coll.Cardiol. 1993;22:514-520.

5. Baumgart D, Haude M, Goerge G et al. Improved assessment of coronary stenosis severity using the relative flow velocity reserve. Circulation 1998;98:40-46.

6. Baumgart D, Haude M, Liu F et al. Current concepts of coronary flow reserve for clinical decision making during cardiac catheterization. Am.Heart J. 1998;136:136-149.

7. Bayliss J, Pearson M, Sutton GC. Ventricular dysrhythmias following intravenous dipyridamole during "stress" myocardial imaging. Br.J.Radiol. 1983;56:669-686.

8. Bech GJ, de Bruyne B, Bonnier HJ et al. Long-term follow-up after deferral of percutaneous transluminal coronary angioplasty of intermediate stenosis on the basis of coronary pressure measurement. J.Am.Coll.Cardiol. 1998;31:841-847.

9. Bech GJ, Droste H, Pijls N et al. Value of fractional flow reserve in making decisions about bypass surgery for equivocal left main coronary artery disease. Heart 2001;86:547-552.

10. Bech GJ, Pijls N, de Bruyne B et al. Usefulness of fractional flow reserve to predict clinical outcome after balloon angioplasty. Circulation 1999;96:883-888.

11. Becher H, Burns PN. Handbook of contrast echocardiography, left ventricular function and myocardial perfusion. Frankfurt and New York: Springer Verlag, 2000.

12. Benchimol D, Mazanof M, Dubroca B et al. Detection of coronary stenoses by stress echocardiography using a previously implanted pacemaker for ventricular pacing: preliminary report of a new method. Clin.Cardiol. 2000;23:842-848.

13.	Benzuly KH, Padgett RC, Kaul S et al. Functional improvement precedes structural regression of atherosclerosis. Circulation 1994;89:1810-1818.

14.	Beręsewicz, A. Regulacja przepywu wieńcowego. In: Januszewicz A, ed. Nadciśnienie tętnicze. Kraków: Medycyna Praktyczna, 2000: 239-244.

15.	Billinger M, Seiler C, Fleisch M et al. Do beta-adrenergic blocking agents increase coronary flow reserve? J.Am.Coll.Cardiol. 2001;38:1866-1871.

16.	Blumenthal MS, McCauley CS. Cardiac arrest during dipyridamole imaging. Chest 1988;93:1103-1104.

17.	Bookstein JJ, Higgins CB. Comparative efficacy of coronary vasodilatory methods. Invest Radiol. 1977;12:121-127.

18.	Bourdarias JP. Coronary reserve: concept and physiological variations. Eur.Heart J. 1995;16 Suppl I:2-6.

19.	Caiati C, Cioglia G, Montaldo C et al. Correlation of 99mTc-sestamibi SPECT myocardial perfusion imaging with absolute coronary flow reserve by a new noninvasive Doppler method in patients with stenoses of the left anterior descending coronary artery. A preliminary report. Cardiologia 1999;44:809-816.

20.	Caiati C, Montaldo C, Zedda N et al. New noninvasive method for coronary flow reserve assessment: contrast- enhanced transthoracic second harmonic echo Doppler. Circulation 1999;99:771-778.

21.	Caiati C, Montaldo C, Zedda N et al. Validation of a new noninvasive method (contrast-enhanced transthoracic second harmonic echo Doppler) for the evaluation of coronary flow reserve: comparison with intracoronary Doppler flow wire. J.Am.Coll.Cardiol. 1999;34:1193-1200.

22.	Caiati C, Zedda N, Montaldo C et al. Contrast-enhanced transthoracic second harmonic echo Doppler with adenosine: a noninvasive, rapid and effective method for coronary flow reserve assessment. J.Am.Coll.Cardiol. 1999;34:122-130.

23.	Campisi R, Czernin J, Schoder H et al. Effects of long-term smoking on myocardial blood flow, coronary vasomotion, and vasodilator capacity. Circulation 1998;98:119-125.

24.	Cannon RO, III. Does coronary endothelial dysfunction cause myocardial ischemia in the absence of obstructive coronary artery disease? Circulation 1997;96:3251-3254.

25.	Cannon RO, III, Curiel RV, Prasad A et al. Comparison of coronary endothelial dynamics with electrocardiographic and left ventricular contractile response to stress in the absence of coronary artery disease. Am.J.Cardiol. 1998;82:710-714.

26.	Cannon RO, III, Rosing DR, Maron BJ et al. Myocardial ischemia in patients with hypertrophic cardiomyopathy: contribution of inadequate vasodilator reserve and elevated left ventricular filling pressures. Circulation 1985;71:234-243.

27.	Cannon RO, III, Schenke WH, Maron BJ et al. Differences in coronary flow and myocardial metabolism at rest and during pacing between patients with obstructive and patients with nonobstructive hypertrophic cardiomyopathy. J.Am.Coll.Cardiol. 1987;10:53-62.

28.	Cecchi F, Gistri R, Olivotto I et al. Impairment of coronary vasodilator capacity is predictive of unfavorable outcome in patients with hypertrophic cardiomyopathy (abstract). Eur.Heart J. 2000;21(Abstract Supplement):257.

29.	Chamuleau SA, Meuwissen M, Eck-Smit BL et al. Fractional flow reserve, absolute and relative coronary blood flow velocity reserve in relation to the results of technetium-99m sestamibi single-photon emission computed tomography in patients with two-vessel coronary artery disease. J.Am.Coll.Cardiol. 2001;37:1316-1322.

30.	Chauhan A, Mullins PA, Petch MC et al. Is coronary flow reserve in response to papaverine really normal in syndrome X? Circulation 1994;89:1998-2004.

31.   Chauhan A, Mullins PA, Taylor MC et al. Both endothelium-dependent and endothelium-independent function is impaired in patients with angina pectoris and normal coronary angiograms. Eur.Heart J. 1997;18:60-68.

32.   Chen K, Colonna P, Cadeddu M et al. Coronary flow reserve is correlated with no-reflow phenomenon and has predictive value of myocardial viability in patients with reperfused acute anterior myocardial infarction (abstract). Circulation 2001;104 (Abstract Supplement):3533.

33.   Chen K, Colonna P, Montisci R et al. Coronary steal detected noninvasively by contrast-enhanced transthoracic harmonic color Doppler echocardiography. (abstract). Eur.Heart J. 2001;22 (Abstract Supp):2812.

34.   Chilian WM. Coronary microcirculation in health and disease. Summary of an NHLBI workshop. Circulation 1997;95:522-528.

35.   Chilian WM, Kuo L, DeFily DV et al. Endothelial regulation of coronary microvascular tone under physiological and pathophysiological conditions. Eur.Heart J. 1993;14 Suppl I:55-59.

36.   Chirillo F, Bruni A, Balestra G et al. Assessment of internal mammary artery and saphenous vein graft patency and flow reserve using transthoracic Doppler echocardiography. Heart 2001;86:424-431.

37.   Choudhury L, Elliott P, Rimoldi O et al. Transmural myocardial blood flow distribution in hypertrophic cardiomyopathy and effect of treatment. Basic Res Cardiol. 1999;94:49-59.

38.   Colonna P, Cadeddu M, Selem AH et al. Preserved coronary flow velocity reserve in patients with acute myocardial infarction and ischemic preconditioning due to preinfarction angina (abstract). Circulation 2001;104 (Abstract Supplement):2169.

39.   Crowley JJ, Dardas PS, Harcombe AA et al. Transthoracic Doppler echocardiographic analysis of phasic coronary blood flow velocity in hypertrophic cardiomyopathy. Heart 1997;77:558-563.

40.   Crowley JJ, Shapiro LM. Transthoracic echocardiographic measurement of coronary blood flow and reserve. J.Am.Soc.Echocardiogr. 1997;10:337-343.

41.   Czernin J, Muller P, Chan S et al. Influence of age and hemodynamics on myocardial blood flow and flow reserve. Circulation 1993;88:62-69.

42.   Daimon M, Watanabe H, Yamagishi H et al. Physiologic assessment of coronary artery stenosis by coronary flow reserve measurements with transthoracic Doppler echocardiography: comparison with exercise thallium-201 single positron emission computed tomography. J.Am.Coll.Cardiol. 2001;37:1310-1315.

43.   De Simone L, Caso P, Severino S. Noninvasive assessment of left and right internal mammary artery graft patency with high frequency transthoracic echocardiography. J.Am.Soc.Echocardiogr. 1999;12:841-849.

44.   Di Carli MF, Bianco-Batlles D, Landa ME et al. Effects of autonomic neuropathy on coronary blood flow in patients with diabetes mellitus. Circulation 1999;100:813-819.

45.   Di Mario C, Moses JW, Anderson TJ et al. Randomized comparison of elective stent implantation and coronary balloon angioplasty guided by online quantitative angiography and intracoronary Doppler. DESTINI Study Group (Doppler Endpoint STenting INternational Investigation). Circulation 2000;102:2938-2944.

46.   Di Segni E, Higano ST, Rihal CS et al. Incremental doses of intracoronary adenosine for the assessment of the coronary velocity reserve for clinical decision making. Catheter.Cardiovasc.Interv. 2001;54:34-40.

47.   Dubois-Rande JL, Dupouy P, Aptecar E et al. Comparison of the effects of exercise and cold pressor test on the vasomotor response of normal and atherosclerotic coronary

arteries and their relation to the flow-mediated mechanism. Am.J.Cardiol. 1995;76:467-473.

48.   Duffy SJ, Gelman JS, Peverill RE et al. Agreement between coronary flow velocity reserve and stress echocardiography in intermediate-severity coronary stenoses. Catheter.Cardiovasc.Interv. 2001;53:29-38.

49.   Dupouy P, Pelle G, Garot P et al. Physiologically guided angioplasty in support to a provisional stenting strategy: immediate and six-month outcome. Catheter.Cardiovasc.Interv. 2000;49:369-375.

50.   El Shafei A, Chiravuri R, Stikovac MM et al. Comparison of relative coronary Doppler flow velocity reserve to stress myocardial perfusion imaging in patients with coronary artery disease. Catheter.Cardiovasc.Interv. 2001;53:193-201.

51.   Feinstein SB, Voci P, Pizzuto F. Nonivasive surrogate markers of atherosclerosis. Am.J.Cardiol. 2002;89(suppl):31C-44C.

52.   Furchgott RF, Zawadzki JV. The obligatory role of endothelial cells in the relaxation of arterial smooth muscle by acetylcholine. Nature 1980;288:373-376.

53.   Fusejima K. Noninvasive measurement of coronary artery blood flow using combined two-dimensional and Doppler echocardiography. J.Am.Coll.Cardiol. 1987;10:1024-1031.

54.   Fusejima K, Takahara Y, Sudo Y et al. Comparison of coronary hemodynamics in patients with internal mammary artery and saphenous vein coronary artery bypass grafts: a noninvasive approach using combined two-dimensional and Doppler echocardiography. J.Am.Coll.Cardiol. 1990;15:131-139.

55.   Ganz, P. and Ganz, W. Coronary blood flow and myocardial ischemia. In: Braunwald E, Zipes DP, Libby P, eds. Heart Disease. W.B.Sauders, 2001: 1087-1113.

56.   Gistri R, Cecchi F, Choudhury L et al. Effect of verapamil on absolute myocardial blood flow in hypertrophic cardiomyopathy. Am.J.Cardiol. 1994;74:363-368.

57.   Globits S, Sakuma H, Shimakawa A et al. Measurement of coronary blood flow velocity during handgrip exercise using breath-hold velocity encoded cine magnetic resonance imaging. Am.J.Cardiol. 1997;79:234-237.

58.   Gordon JB, Ganz P, Nabel EG et al. Atherosclerosis influences the vasomotor response of epicardial coronary arteries to exercise. J.Clin.Invest 1989;83:1946-1952.

59.   Gould KL, Kirkeeide RL, Buchi M. Coronary flow reserve as a physiologic measure of stenosis severity. J.Am.Coll.Cardiol. 1990;15:459-474.

60.   Gould KL, Lipscomb K, Hamilto GW. Physiology basis for assessing critical coronary stenosis: instantaneous flow response and regional distribution during coronary hyperemia as measures of coronary flow reserve. Am.J.Cardiol. 1974;33:87-94.

61.   Gould KL, Martucci JP, Goldberg DI. Short-term cholesterol lowering decreases in size and severity of perfusion abnormalities by positron emission tomography after dipyridamole in patients with coronary artery disease. Circulation 1994;89:1530-1538.

62.   Hasdai D, Gibbons RJ, Holmes DR, Jr. et al. Coronary endothelial dysfunction in humans is associated with myocardial perfusion defects. Circulation 1997;96:3390-3395.

63.   Hasdai D, Holmes DR, Jr., Higano ST et al. Prevalence of coronary blood flow reserve abnormalities among patients with nonobstructive coronary artery disease and chest pain. Mayo Clin.Proc. 1998;73:1133-1140.

64.   Haude M, Baumgart D, Verna E et al. Intracoronary Doppler- and quantitative coronary angiography derived predictors of major adverse cardiac events after stent implantation. Circulation 2001;103:1212-1217.

65.   Haude M, Herrmann J, Baumgart D et al. Absolute and relative coronary flow velocity reserve for discrimination between acute periinterventional and chronic

poststenotic microvascular disorders. (abstract). Eur.Heart J. 2001;22 (Abstract Supplement):473.

66.   Haynes WG, Ferro CJ, O'Kane KP et al. Systemic endothelin receptor blockade decreases peripheral vascular resistance and blood pressure in humans. Circulation 1996;93:1860-1870.

67.   Herrmann J, Haude M, Lerman A et al. Abnormal coronary flow velocity reserve after coronary intervention is associated with cardiac marker elevation. Circualtion 2001;103:2339-2345.

68.   Higashiue S, Watanabe H, Yokoi Y et al. Simple detection of severe coronary stenosis using transthoracic doppler echocardiography at rest. Am.J.Cardiol. 2001;87:1064-1068.

69.   Hildick-Smith DJ, Johnson PJ, Wisbey CR et al. Coronary flow reserve is supranormal in endurance athletes: an adenosine transthoracic echocardiographic study. Heart 2000;84:383-389.

70.   Hildick-Smith DJ, Shapiro LM. Transthoracic echocardiographic measurement of coronary artery diameter: validation against quantitative coronary angiography. J.Am.Soc.Echocardiogr. 1998;11:893-897.

71.   Hildick-Smith DJ, Shapiro LM. Coronary flow reserve improves after aortic valve replacement for aortic stenosis: an adenosine transthoracic echocardiography study. J.Am.Coll.Cardiol. 2000;36:1889-1896.

72.   Hirata K, Shimada K, Watanabe H et al. Modulation of coronary flow velocity reserve by gender, menstrual cycle and hormone replacement therapy. J.Am.Coll.Cardiol. 2001;38:1879-1884.

73.   Hirata K, Watanabe H, Takai KJr et al. The value of reverse diastolic flow for the presence of occluded coronary artery: Noninvasive detection by transthoracic Doppler echocardigraphy (abstract). Circulation 2001;104 (Abstract Supplement):2345.

74.   Hoffman JI. Problems of coronary flow reserve. Ann.Biomed.Eng 2000;28:884-896.

75.   Holdright DR, Lindsay DC, Clarke D et al. Coronary flow reserve in patients with chest pain and normal coronary arteries. Br.Heart J. 1993;70:513-519.

76.   Houghton JL, Smith VE, Breisblatt WM et al. Coronary vasomotor function in a normotensive, nondiabetic referral population with normal coronary arteriograms. Am.J.Cardiol. 1996;77:1241-1244.

77.   Hozumi T, Eisenberg M, Sugioka K et al. Change in coronary flow reserve on transthoracic Doppler echocardiography after a single high-fat meal in young healthy men. Ann Inter Med 2002;136:523-528.

78.   Hozumi T, Yoshida K, Akasaka T et al. Value of acceleration flow and the prestenotic to stenotic coronary flow velocity ratio by transthoracic color Doppler echocardiography in noninvasive diagnosis of restenosis after percutaneous transluminal coronary angioplasty. J.Am.Coll.Cardiol. 2000;35:164-168.

79.   Hozumi T, Yoshida K, Ogata Y et al. Noninvasive assessment of significant left anterior descending coronary artery stenosis by coronary flow velocity reserve with transthoracic color Doppler echocardiography. Circulation 1998;97:1557-1562.

80.   Huggins GS, Pasternak RC, Alpert NM et al. Effect of short term treatment of hyperlipidemia on coronary vasodilator function and myocardial perfusion in regions having substantial impairment of baseline dilator reserve. Circulation 1998;98:1291-1296.

81.   Iida H, Fujii T, Miura T et al. Assessment of endothelium dependent coronary vasodilation in hypertrophic cardiomyopathy. (abstract). Circulation 1996;94 (Abstract Supplement):I-502.

82.   Iida H, Yokoyama I, Agostini D et al. Quantitative assessment of regional myocardial blood flow using oxygen- 15-labelled water and positron emission tomography: a multicentre evaluation in Japan. Eur.J.Nucl.Med. 2000;27:192-201.

83.   Ishihara M, Sato H, Tateishi H et al. Effects of various doses of intracoronary verapamil on coronary resistance vessels in humans. Jpn.Circ J. 1997;61:755-761.

84.   Johnson PC. Autoregulation of blood flow. Circ Res 1986;59:483-495.

85.   Jones CJ, Kuo L, Davis MJ et al. Distribution and control of coronary microvascular resistance. Adv.Exp.Med.Biol. 1993;346:181-188.

86.   Jones CJ, Kuo L, Davis MJ et al. Myogenic and flow-dependent control mechanisms in the coronary microcirculation. Basic Res.Cardiol. 1993;88:2-10.

87.   Joye JD, Schulman DS, Lasorda D et al. Intracoronary Doppler guide wire versus stress single-photon emission computed tomographic thallium-201 imaging in assessment of intermediate coronary stenoses. J.Am.Coll.Cardiol. 1994;24:940-947.

88.   Kasprzak JD, Drożdż J, Peruga JZ et al. Doppler detection of proximal coronary artery stenosis using transesophageal echocardiography. Kardiol Pol 1999;50:491-500.

89.   Kasprzak JD, Drożdż J, Peruga JZ et al. Definition of flow parameters in proximal nonstenotic coronary arteries using transesophageal Doppler echocardiography. Echocardiography. 2000;17:141-150.

90.   Kasprzak JD, Krzemińska-Pakula M, Drożdż J et al. Transesophageal echocardiographic assessment of proximal coronary flow: definition of normal values. Kardiol Pol 1997;47:208-214.

91.   Kenny A, Shapiro LM. Transthoracic high-frequency two-dimensional echocardiography, Doppler and color flow mapping to determine anatomy and blood flow patterns in the distal left anterior descending coronary artery. Am.J.Cardiol. 1992;69:1265-1268.

92.   Kern MJ. Coronary physiology revisited: practical insights from the cardiac catheterization laboratory. Circulation 2000;101:1344-1351.

93.   Kern MJ, Bach RG, Mechem CJ et al. Variations in normal coronary vasodilatory reserve stratified by artery, gender, heart transplantation and coronary artery disease. J.Am.Coll.Cardiol. 1996;28:1154-1160.

94.   Kern MJ, de Bruyne B, Pijls N. From research to clinical practice: current role of physiologically based decision making in the catheterization laboratory. J.Am.Coll.Cardiol. 1997;30:613-620.

95.   Kern MJ, Hodgson JM, Rossen JD. Hyperemic coronary blood flow induced by selective adenosine A_{2A} receptor stimulation: first report in patients of a well tolerated novel agent for stress imaging (abstract). J.Am.Coll.Cardiol. 2001;37(Abstract Supplement):299.

96.   Kimball BP, LiPreti V, Bui S et al. Comparison of proximal left anterior descending and circumflex coronary artery dimensions in aortic valve stenosis and hypertrophic cardiomyopathy. Am.J.Cardiol. 1990;65:767-771.

97.   Klocke FJ. Clinical and experimental evaluations of the functional severity of coronary stenoses. Newsletter of the Council on Clinical Cardiology of the AHA, Inc. 1982;7:1-9.

98.   Klocke FJ. Measurements of coronary flow reserve: defining pathophysiology versus making decisions about patient care. Circulation 1987;76:1183-1189.

99.   Kodama K, Hamada M, Kazatani Y et al. Clinical characteristics in Japanese patients with coexistence of hypertrophic cardiomyopathy and coronary vasospasm. Angiology 1998;49:849-855.

100. Kofoed KF, Czernin J, Johnson J et al. Effects of cardiac allograft vasculopathy on myocardial blood flow, vasodilatory capacity, and coronary vasomotion. Circulation 1997;95:600-606.

101. Kozakova M, Palombo C, Pratali L et al. Mechanisms of coronary flow reserve impairment in human hypertension. An integrated approach by transthoracic and transesophageal echocardiography. Hypertension 1997;29:551-559.

102. Krams R, Kofflard MJ, Duncker DJ et al. Decreased coronary flow reserve in hypertrophic cardiomyopathy is related to remodeling of the coronary microcirculation. Circulation 1998;97:230-233.

103. Krzanowski M, Bodzon W, Brzostek T et al. Value of transthoracic echocardiography for the detection of high-grade coronary artery stenosis: prospective evaluation in 50 consecutive patients scheduled for coronary angiography. J.Am.Soc.Echocardiogr. 2000;13:1091-1099.

104. Kyriakidis MK, Dernellis JM, Androulakis AE et al. Changes in phasic coronary blood flow velocity profile and relative coronary flow reserve in patients with hypertrophic obstructive cardiomyopathy. Circulation 1997;96:834-841.

105. Lambertz H, Tries HP, Stein T et al. Noninvasive assessment of coronary flow reserve with transthoracic signal-enhanced Doppler echocardiography. J.Am.Soc.Echocardiogr. 1999;12:186-195.

106. Lee CY, Pellikka PA, McCully RB et al. Nonexercise stress transthoracic echocardiography: transesophageal atrial pacing versus dobutamine stress. J.Am.Coll.Cardiol. 1999;33:506-511.

107. Lethen H, Tries HP, Kersting S et al. Transthoracic echocardiography measurement of coronary flow reserve in the right coronary artery: comparison with invasive data (abstract). J.Am.Coll.Cardiol. 2002;39 (Abstract Supplement):1045-61.

108. Lewen MK, Labovitz AJ, Kern MJ et al. Prolonged myocardial ischemia after intravenous dipyridamole thallium imaging. Chest 1987;92:1102-1104.

109. Lim HE, Shim WJ, Rhee H et al. Assessment of coronary flow reserve with transthoracic Doppler echocardiography: comparison among adenosine, standard-dose dipyridamole, and high-dose dipyridamole. J.Am.Soc.Echocardiogr. 2000;13:264-270.

110. Lorenzoni R, Gistri R, Cecchi F et al. Coronary vasodilator reserve is impaired in patients with hypertrophic cardiomyopathy and left ventricular dysfunction. Am.Heart J. 1998;136:972-981.

111. Lowenstein J, Presti C, Tiano C. Noninvasive assessment of coronary flow reserve by transthoracic Doppler echocardiography in a general referral population: experience on 957 patients (abstract). Eur.Heart J. 2001;22(Abstract Supplement):347.

112. Ludmer PL, Selwyn AP, Shook TL et al. Paradoxical vasoconstriction induced by acetylcholine in atherosclerotic coronary arteries. N.Engl.J.Med. 1986;315:1046-1051.

113. Luscher TF, Barton M. Biology of the endothelium. Clin.Cardiol. 1997;20:II-10.

114. Maczewski M, Beręsewicz A. Metody czynnościowe oceny funkcji śródbłonka naczyniowego. Kardiol Pol 1998;48:50-56.

115. Marcus ML, White CW. Coronary flow reserve in patients with normal coronary angiograms. J.Am.Coll.Cardiol. 1985;6:1254-1256.

116. Maron BJ, Wolfson JK, Epstein SE et al. Intramural ("small vessel") coronary artery disease in hypertrophic cardiomyopathy. J.Am.Coll.Cardiol. 1986;8:545-557.

117. Masuda D, Nohara R, Tamaki N et al. Evaluation of coronary blood flow reserve by 13N-NH3 positron emission computed tomography (PET) with dipyridamole in the treatment of hypertension with the ACE inhibitor (Cilazapril). Ann.Nucl.Med. 2000;14:353-360.

118. Mazeika P, Nihoyannopoulos P, Joshi J et al. Uses and limitations of high dose dipyridamole stress echocardiography for evaluation of coronary artery disease. Br.Heart J. 1992;67:144-149.

119. McGinn AL, White CW, Wilson RF. Interstudy variability of coronary flow reserve. Influence of heart rate, arterial pressure, and ventricular preload. Circulation 1990;81:1319-1330.

120. McLenachan JM, Williams JK, Fish RD et al. Loss of flow-mediated endothelium-dependent dilation occurs early in the development of atherosclerosis. Circulation 1991;84:1273-1278.

121. Meeder JG, Peels HO, Blanksma PK. Comparison between positron emission tomography myocardial perfusion imaging and intracoronary Doppler flow velocity measurements at acetylcholine and during cold pressor testing in angiographically normal coronary arteries in patients with one-vessel coronary artery disease. Am.J.Cardiol. 1996;78:526-531.

122. Memmola C, Iliceto S, Napoli VF et al. Coronary flow dynamics and reserve assessed by transesophageal echocardiography in obstructive hypertrophic cardiomyopathy. Am.J.Cardiol. 1994;74:1147-1151.

123. Miller DD, Donohue TJ, Younis LT et al. Correlation of pharmacological 99mTc-sestamibi myocardial perfusion imaging with poststenotic coronary flow reserve in patients with angiographically intermediate coronary artery stenoses. Circulation 1994;89:2150-2160.

124. Miyazaki C, Takeuchi K, Yoshitani H et al. Assessment of the reduction of coronary flow velocity reserve in patients with diabetic retinopathy by transthoracic Doppler echocardiography (abstract). J.Am.Coll.Cardiol. 2002;39 (Abstract Supplement):1045-60.

125. Miyazaki C, Takeuchi K, Yoshitani H et al. The optimum hypoglycemic therapy can improve coronary flow velocity reserve in diabetic patients: demonstration by transthoracic Doppler echocardiography (abstract). J.Am.Coll.Cardiol. 2002;39 (Abstract Supplement):1045-59.

126. Mombouli JV, Vanhoutte PM. Endothelial dysfunction: from physiology to therapy. J.Mol.Cell Cardiol. 1999;31:61-74.

127. Mosher PJ, Ross JrJ, McFate PA et al. Control of coronary blood flow by an autoregulatory mechanism. Circ Res 1964;14:250-259.

128. Nabel EG, Ganz P, Gordon JB et al. Dilation of normal and constriction of atherosclerotic coronary arteries caused by the cold pressor test. Circulation 1988;77:43-52.

129. Nabel EG, Selwyn AP, Ganz P. Paradoxical narrowing of atherosclerotic coronary arteries induced by increases in heart rate. Circulation 1990;81:850-859.

130. Nasu T, Yashima N, Kuriki S et al. Diagnosis of restenosis after coronary intervention to left coronary artery lesion by transthoracic Doppler coronary echo.(abstract). Circulation 1998;98 (Abstract Supplement):I-163.

131. Ochala A, Sanecki P, Gabrylewicz B et al. The use of contrast-enhanced transthoracic second harmonic echo Doppler for noninvasive assessment of coronary angioplasty results.(abstract). Eur.Heart J. 2001;22 (Abstract Supplement):346.

132. Ochala A, Tendera M, Poloński L et al. Mechanism responsible for angina pectoris in hypertrophic cardiomyopathy. Kardiol Pol 1995;42:364-368.

133. Otsuka R, Watanabe H, Hirata K et al. Acute effects of passive smoking on the coronary circulation in healthy young adults. JAMA 2001;286:436-441.

134. Otsuka R, Watanabe H, Kumiko H et al. Simple detection of the occluded right coronary artery using thransthoracic echocardiography at rest (abstract). Circulation 2001;104 (Abstract Supplement):3175.

135. Parodi O, Neglia D, Palombo C et al. Comparative effects of enalapril and verapamil on myocardial blood flow in systemic hypertension. Circulation 1997;96:864-873.

136. Petkow-Dimitrow P, Krzanowski M, Bodzon W et al. Coronary flow reserve and exercise capacity in hypertrophic cardiomyopathy. Heart Vessels 1996;11:160-164.

137. Petkow-Dimitrow P, Krzanowski M, Grodecki.J et al. Verapamil improves the endothelium-dependent vasodilatation in patients with hypertrophic cardiomyopathy. International J Cardiol 2002;83:239-47.

138. Petkow-Dimitrow P, Krzanowski M, Niżankowski R et al. Verapamil improves the response of coronary vasomotion to cold pressor test in asymptomatic and mildly symptomatic patients with hypertrophic cardiomyopathy. Cardiovasc.Drugs Ther. 1999;13:259-264.

139. Petkow-Dimitrow P, Krzanowski M, Niżankowski R et al. Comparison of the effect of verapamil and propranolol on response of coronary vasomotion to cold pressor test in symptomatic patients with hypertrophic cardiomyopathy. Cardiovasc.Drugs Ther. 2000;14:643-650.

140. Petkow-Dimitrow P, Krzanowski M, Niżankowski R et al. Effect of verapamil on systolic and diastolic coronary blood flow velocity in asymptomatic and mildly symptomatic patients with hypertrophic cardiomyopathy. Heart 2000;83:262-266.

141. Petkow-Dimitrow P, Krzanowski M, Niżankowski R et al. The effect of verapamil on response of coronary vasomotory to handgrip exercise in symptomatic patients with hypertrophic cardiomyopathy. Cardiovasc.Drugs Ther. 2001;15:331-337.

142. Petkow-Dimitrow P, Krzanowski M, Zdzienicka A et al. Elevated endothelin concentrations are associated with reduced coronary vasomotor response to exercise in patients with hypertrophic cardiomyopathy. (abstract). Eur.Heart J. 2001;22 (Abstract Supplement):408.

143. Petkow-Dimitrow P, Surdacki A, Dubiel JS. Verapamil normalizes the response of left ventricular early diastolic filling to cold pressor test in asymptomatic and mildly symptomatic patients with hypertophic cardiomyopathy. Cardiovasc.Drugs Ther. 1997;11:741-746.

144. Piek JJ, Boersma E, Di Mario C et al. Angiographical and Doppler flow-derived parameters for assessment of coronary lesion severity and its relation to the result of exercise electrocardiography. DEBATE study group. Doppler Endpoints Balloon Angioplasty Trial Europe. Eur.Heart J. 2000;21:466-474.

145. Pijls NH, de Bruyne B, Peels K et al. Measurement of fractional flow reserve to assess the functional severity of coronary-artery stenoses. N.Engl.J.Med. 1996;334:1703-1708.

146. Pizzuto F, Voci P, Mariano E et al. Assessment of flow velocity reserve by transthoracic Doppler echocardiography and venous adenosine infusion before and after left anterior descending coronary artery stenting. J.Am.Coll.Cardiol. 2001;38:155-162.

147. Quyyumi AA, Dakak N, Andrews NP et al. Contribution of nitric oxide to metabolic coronary vasodilation in the human heart. Circulation 1995;92:320-326.

148. Quyyumi AA, Dakak N, Andrews NP et al. Nitric oxide activity in the human coronary circulation. Impact of risk factors for coronary atherosclerosis. J.Clin.Invest 1995;95:1747-1755.

149. Radvan J, Marwick TH, Williams MJ et al. Evaluation of the extent and timing of the coronary hyperemic response to dipyridamole: a study with transesophageal echocardiography and positron emission tomography with oxygen 15 water. J.Am.Soc.Echocardiogr. 1995;8:864-873.

150. Reis SE, Holubkov R, Lee JS et al. Coronary flow velocity response to adenosine characterizes coronary microvascular function in women with chest pain and no obstructive coronary disease. Results from the pilot phase of the Women's Ischemia Syndrome Evaluation (WISE) study. J.Am.Coll.Cardiol. 1999;33:1469-1475.

151. Rigo F, Curtaia W, Zanella C et al. Noninvasive assessment of left anterior descending artery coronary flow reserve by transthoracic echocardiography: feasibility and results (abstract). J.Am.Coll.Cardiol. 2002;39 (Abstract Supplement):1164-60.

152. Ross JJ, Jr., Mintz GS, Chandrasekaran K. Transthoracic two-dimensional high frequency (7.5 MHz) ultrasonic visualization of the distal left anterior descending coronary artery. J.Am.Coll.Cardiol. 1990;15:373-377.

153. Rossen JD, Nahser PJ, Jr., Oskarsson H et al. Does pharmacologic coronary flow reserve reflect vasodilator responsiveness to increased myocardial demand in humans? Coron.Artery Dis. 1996;7:479-484.

154. Rossen JD, Quillen JE, Lopez AG et al. Comparison of coronary vasodilation with intravenous dipyridamole and adenosine. J.Am.Coll.Cardiol. 1991;18:485-491.

155. Rossen JD, Winniford MD. Effect of increases in heart rate and arterial pressure on coronary flow reserve in humans. J.Am.Coll.Cardiol. 1993;21:343-348.

156. Sambuceti G, Marzilli M, Marraccini P et al. Coronary vasoconstriction during myocardial ischemia induced by rises in metabolic demand in patients with coronary artery disease. Circulation 1997;95:2652-2659.

157. Saraste M, Koskenvuo J, Knuuti J et al. Coronary flow reserve: measurement with transthoracic Doppler echocardiography is reproducible and comparable with positron emission tomography. Clin.Physiol 2001;21:114-122.

158. Saraste M, Koskenvuo JW, Mikkola J et al. Technical achievement: transthoracic Doppler echocardiography can be used to detect LAD restenosis after coronary angioplasty. Clin.Physiol 2000;20:428-433.

159. Schachinger V, Britten MB, Zeiher AM. Prognostic impact of coronary vasodilator dysfunction on adverse long-term outcome of coronary heart disease. Circulation 2000;101:1899-1906.

160. Schachinger V, Zeiher AM. Prognostic implications of endothelial dysfunction: does it mean anything? Coron.Artery Dis. 2001;12:435-443.

161. Schelbert HR. Positron emission tomography and the changing paradigm in coronary artery disease. Z Kardiol 2000;89 Suppl 4:IV55-66.

162. Schwartzkopff B, Mundhenke M, Strauer BE. Alterations of the architecture of subendocardial arterioles in patients with hypertrophic cardiomyopathy and impaired coronary vasodilator reserve: a possible cause for myocardial ischemia. J.Am.Coll.Cardiol. 1998;31:1089-1096.

163. Serruys PW, de Bruyne B, Carlier S et al. Randomized comparison of primary stenting and provisional balloon angioplasty guided by flow velocity measurement. Doppler Endpoints Balloon Angioplasty Trial Europe (DEBATE) II Study Group. Circulation 2000;102:2930-2937.

164. Serruys PW, Di Mario C, Piek J et al. Prognostic value of intracoronary flow velocity and diameter stenosis in assessing the stenosis in assessing the short- and long-term outcomes of coronary balloon angioplasty; the DEBATE study. Circulation 1997;96:3369-3377.

165. Smith TP, Jr., Canty JM, Jr. Modulation of coronary autoregulatory responses by nitric oxide. Evidence for flow-dependent resistance adjustments in conscious dogs. Circ Res 1993;73:232-240.

166. Steinberg HO, Tarshoby M, Monestel R et al. Elevated circulating free fatty acid levels impair endothelium- dependent vasodilation. J.Clin.Invest 1997;100:1230-1239.

167. Stepp DW, Nishikawa Y, Chilian WM. Regulation of shear stress in the canine coronary microcirculation. Circulation 1999;100:1555-1561.

168. Sudhir K, MacGregor JS, Gupta M et al. Effect of selective angiotensin II receptor antagonism and angiotensin converting enzyme inhibition on the coronary vasculature in vivo. Intravascular two-dimensional and Doppler ultrasound studies. Circulation 1993;87:931-938.

169. Suwaidi J, Hamasaki S, Higano ST et al. Long-term follow-up of patients with mild coronary artery disease and endothelial dysfunction. Circulation 2000;101:948-954.

170. Suzuki H, Koba S, Takeyama Y et al. Ultrastructural changes of blood capillaries in patients with microvascular angina, hypertrophic cardiomyopathy, and dilated cardiomyopathy. Am J Cardiovasc Pathol 1995;5:15-26.

171. Tadamura E, Iida H, Matsumoto K et al. Comparison of myocardial blood flow during dobutamine-atropine infusion with that after dipyridamole administartion in normal men. J.Am.Coll.Cardiol. 2001;37:130-136.

172. Tadamura E, Yoshbayashi M, Yonemura T et al. Significant regional heterogeneity of coronary flow reserve in paediatric hypertrophic cardiomyopathy. Eur.J.Nucl.Med. 2000;27:1340-1348.

173. Takemura G, Takatsu Y, Fujiwara H. Luminal narrowing of coronary capillaries in human hypertrophic hearts: An ultrastructural morphometrical study using endomyocardial biopsy specimens. Heart 1998;78-85.

174. Takeuchi M, Miyazaki C, Yoshitani H et al. Assessment of coronary flow velocity with transthoracic Doppler echocardiography during dobutamine stress echocardiography. J.Am.Coll.Cardiol. 2001;38:117-123.

175. Tamai O, Matsuoka H, Itabe H et al. Single LDL apheresis improves endothelium-dependent vasodilatation in hypercholesterolemic humans. Circulation 1997;95:76-82.

176. Tanaka M, Fujiwara M, Onodera T et al. Quantitative analysis of narrowings of intramyocardial small arteries in normal hearts, hypertensive hearts, and hearts with hypertophic cardiomyopathy. Circulation 1987;75:1130-1139.

177. Tokai K, Watanabe H, Yamagishi H et al. Noninvasive diagnosis of physiologic stenosis in the left circumflex coronary artery using contrast enhanced transthoracic Doppler echocardiography: comparison with exercise 201-Tl single photon emission computed tomography (abstract). J.Am.Coll.Cardiol. 2002;39 (Abstract Supplement):1094-67.

178. Udelson JE, Bonow RO, O'Gara PT et al. Verapamil prevents silent myocardial perfusion abnormalities during exercise in asymptomatic patients with hypertrophic cardiomyopathy. Circulation 1989;79:1052-1060.

179. Ueda K, Yoshida K, Hozumi T et al. Assessment of restenosis after coronary intervention in the left anterior descending coronary artery by coronary flow velocity reserve determined by transthoracic Doppler echocardiography. (abstract). Circualtion 1998;98 (Abstract Supplement):I-161.

180. Ueno Y, Nakamura T, Kinoshita M. An early predictor of left ventricular remodeling after reperfused anterior acute myocardial infarction: coronary flow velocity reserve with transthoracic Doppler echocardiography (abstract). Circulation 2001;104 (Abstract Supplement):2348.

181. Uren NG, Camici PG, Melin JA et al. Effect of aging on myocardial perfusion reserve. J.Nucl.Med. 1995;36:2032-2036.

182. Uren NG, Crake T, Lefroy DC et al. Delayed recovery of coronary resistive vessel function after coronary angioplasty. J.Am.Coll.Cardiol. 1993;21:612-621.

183. Vallance P, Chan N. Endothelial function and nitric oxide: clinical relevance. Heart 2001;85:342-350.

184. Vane JR, Anggard EE, Botting RM. Regulatory functions of the vascular endothelium. N.Engl.J.Med. 1990;323:27-36.

185. Vassalli G, Hess OM. Measurement of coronary flow reserve and its role in patient care. Basic Res Cardiol. 1998;93:339-353.

186. Ventura HO, Mehra MR, Smart FW et al. Cardiac allograft vasculopathy: current concepts. Am.Heart J. 1995;129:791-798.

187. Verberne HJ, Piek JJ, van Liebergen RA et al. Functional assessment of coronary artery stenosis by Doppler derived absolute and relative coronary blood flow velocity reserve in comparison with (99m)Tc MIBI SPECT. Heart 1999;82:509-514.

188. Verna E, Ceriani L, Giovanella L et al. "False-positive" myocardial perfusion scintigraphy findings in patients with angiographically normal coronary arteries: insights from intravascular sonography studies. J.Nucl.Med. 2000;41:1935-1940.

189. Voci P, Pizzuto F. Coronary flow: How far can we go with echocardiography? J.Am.Coll.Cardiol. 2001;38:1885-1887.

190. Voci P, Testa G, Plaustro G. Imaging of the distal left anterior descending coronary artery by transthoracic color-Doppler echocardiography. Am.J.Cardiol. 1998;81:74G-78G.

191. Vogel RA. Coronary risk factors, endothelial function, and atherosclerosis: a review. Clin.Cardiol. 1997;20:426-432.

192. Watanabe N, Yamaura Y, Akiyama M et al. Noninvasive measurements of coronary collateral flow velocity using transthoracic Doppler echocardiography (abstract). J.Am.Coll.Cardiol. 2002;39 (Abstract Supplement):1164-66.

193. Werns SW, Walton JA, Hsia HH et al. Evidence of endothelial dysfunction in angiographically normal coronary arteries of patients with coronary artery disease. Circulation 1989;79:287-291.

194. White CW, Wright CB, Doty DB et al. Does visual interpretation of the coronary arteriogram predict the physiologic importance of a coronary stenosis? N.Engl.J.Med. 1984;310:819-824.

195. Wilson RF, Laughlin DE, Ackell PH. Transluminal subselective measurement of coronary artery flow velocity and vasodilator reserve in man. Circulation 1985;72:82-92.

196. Yao J, Taams MA, Kasprzak JD et al. Usefulness of three-dimensional transesophageal echocardiographic imaging for evaluating narrowing in the coronary arteries. Am.J.Cardiol. 1999;84:41-45.

197. Yeung AC, Vekshtein VI, Krantz DS et al. The effect of atherosclerosis on the vasomotor response of coronary arteries to mental stress. N.Engl.J.Med. 1991;325:1551-1556.

198. Zeiher AM, Drexler H, Wollschlaeger H et al. Coronary vasomotion in response to sympathetic stimulation in humans: importance of the functional integrity of the endothelium. J.Am.Coll.Cardiol. 1989;14:1181-1190.

199. Zeiher AM, Drexler H, Wollschlager H et al. Endothelial dysfunction of the coronary microvasculature is associated with coronary blood flow regulation in patients with early atherosclerosis. Circulation 1991;84:1984-1992.

200. Zeiher AM, Drexler H, Wollschlager H et al. Modulation of coronary vasomotor tone in humans. Progressive endothelial dysfunction with different early stages of coronary atherosclerosis. Circulation 1991;83:391-401.

201. Zeiher AM, Krause T, Schachinger V et al. Impaired endothelium-dependent vasodilation of coronary resistance vessels is associated with exercise-induced myocardial ischemia. Circulation 1995;91:2345-2352.

INDEX